MW00439443

Yoga, Inc.

Yoga, Inc.

A JOURNEY THROUGH THE BIG BUSINESS OF YOGA

John Philp

Namaste!

March '09

VIKING
CANADA

VIKING CANADA

Published by the Penguin Group

Penguin Group (Canada), 90 Eglinton Avenue East, Suite 700, Toronto, Ontario,
Canada M4P 2Y3 (a division of Pearson Canada Inc.)

Penguin Group (USA) Inc., 375 Hudson Street, New York,
New York 10014, U.S.A.
Penguin Books Ltd, 80 Strand, London WC2R 0RL, England
Penguin Ireland, 25 St Stephen's Green, Dublin 2, Ireland
(a division of Penguin Books Ltd)
Penguin Group (Australia), 250 Camberwell Road, Camberwell, Victoria 3124,
Australia (a division of Pearson Australia Group Pty Ltd)
Penguin Books India Pvt Ltd, 11 Community Centre, Panchsheel Park,
New Delhi – 110 017, India
Penguin Group (NZ), 67 Apollo Drive, Rosedale, North Shore 0632,
New Zealand (a division of Pearson New Zealand Ltd)
Penguin Books (South Africa) (Pty) Ltd, 24 Sturdee Avenue, Rosebank,
Johannesburg 2196, South Africa

Penguin Books Ltd, Registered Offices: 80 Strand, London WC2R 0RL, England

First published 2009

1 2 3 4 5 6 7 8 9 10 (RRD)

Copyright © John Philp, 2009

Manufactured in the U.S.A.

Library and Archives Canada Cataloguing in Publication data available upon
request to the publisher.

ISBN: 978-0-760-06843-2

Visit the Penguin Group (Canada) website at **www.penguin.ca**

Special and corporate bulk purchase rates available; please see
www.penguin.ca/corporatesales or call 1-800-810-3104, ext. 477 or 474

For Goof, Ding, Beatbox and Lisa Jeanne

CONTENTS

INTRODUCTION

Study Yoga; you will learn an infinite amount
from it—but do not try to apply it, for we
Europeans are not so constituted that we apply
these methods correctly, just like that.
—CARL JUNG, *YOGA AND THE WEST*

Some day in the not-too-distant future you're channel surfing on your extra-wide-screen TV and happen to catch the familiar Olympics theme music. Your attention is caught by the triumphant refrain, flashy graphics and rapid-fire visuals. It's the typical athlete profile: our subject psyching himself up, in the heat of battle, thrusting a gold cup aloft. But Esak Garcia isn't a boxer or weightlifter or sprinter. He's a competitive yogi, and he's about to defend his World Olympic Yoga Champion title—after this quick word from Esak's sponsor.

Wait a minute. Competitive yoga? Sponsors? Is this parody or prophecy? You're forgiven for being confused. There really is a competitive yoga circuit, and Esak really has been World Yoga Champion. He doesn't have an endorsement deal, but that's not because he hasn't tried. And while yoga hasn't made it to the Olympics yet, it could just be a matter of time.

Yoga is no longer a mere panacea for the stunning spectrum of physical, mental and spiritual ailments that plague us. Today yoga nets its practitioners gold cups and cash prizes. Yoga is the centerpiece of costly intellectual property lawsuits. Yoga has become the prize in a cross-cultural tug-of-war. Everyone wants a piece of yoga. The unique societal evolution that has led to yoga's exalted position in Western society has been well documented. Less well understood is the central irony that has fueled yoga's spectacular success. The fact is, the further we've blown yoga off its original course, the more we've fed its spectacular success. And it could have happened only here, in the Wild West.

Up against the clock and cursed by an incessant drive to achieve, we have been heading toward epidemic levels of burnout and exhaustion for decades. And in our neurotic, narcoleptic search for peace, we long ago (longer than you probably think) settled on yoga as our spiritual balm. But we want yoga our way. If one factor can be said to define the Western lifestyle, it's convenience. We love the easy answer—the pill that makes you thin, the frying pan that cleans itself, the new car that sweetens your marriage. Our hunger for quick cure-alls soon stretched yoga way beyond the realm of the metaphysical. In short order yoga became detox, rehab, workout and, now, sport. The practice of prayerful meditation is mostly a memory. Hippies and love-ins have been left in the dust. And the celebrity-driven, corporate-backed, body-obsessed, high-priced workout we're left with has purists scratching their heads and asking, Is nothing sacred?

This book is not an attack on yoga itself. Yoga is a discipline, a practice, and any complaints I lodge, no matter how strident, won't change that. It would be like attacking the weather. Besides, yoga isn't mandatory, despite what seems like increasing societal pressure to make it so. If you don't think you'll benefit from this particular system of beliefs, then don't adopt it. Nor is this book an attack on capitalism, big business, entrepreneurship, self-promotion, personal growth, mystical hierarchies of the search for enlightenment. There are no specific prohibitions in the yogic screeds regarding the accumulation of accolades, the reaping of cold, hard cash or the desire for a "sexy back." The sacred scrolls do not *require* you to become enlightened. At its best yoga should, in the parlance of its ardent preachers, "meet you where you are." It should be resilient enough to roll with the seeker, the thinker and the fitness freak. After all, if we can't count on yoga to be flexible, where do we turn?

What this book *does* concern itself with, however, is the gap between saying and doing. If anything, this book has the wholly unoriginal intent of highlighting hypocrisies, only this time our arena is the big business of yoga. This book is about preaching a yogic gospel of renunciation while sizing up suckers for "yoga shoes." It's about slapping your brand name on something that existed before your great-great-grandmother even liked boys. It's about being told to turn inward when our warring, divided world needs our undivided attention. It's about the Big Boys buying up the little boys so they can call themselves Little Boys. It's about the Rowdy West and the Mysterious East, cherry-picked principles and forked tongues, guilelessness and greed.

Why take on yoga, given that it works so well? (Depending on your goals. Taut bellies are within reach. Spiritual transcendence may take more time.) Yoga people are, by and large, an agreeable lot. They certainly proclaim their happiness often enough, and there's no reason to doubt them. So why go after yoga? Because for too long yoga has drifted by on a cushion of good vibes, as if the entire enterprise was somehow above reproach. In the meantime yoga has become monumentally cluttered with all sorts of gimmickry, claptrap and doublespeak that have absolutely nothing to do with the practice itself. All that pseudo-spiritual, biodegradable, emptyheaded, self-serving, Tuvan-throat-singing, back-tatt-sporting, lotus-land, white person post-punk-social-protest hooey that passes for the yoga "lifestyle" has some of us ready to drown a dolphin or torture a pixie.

Think of this book as an antidote to all that. It's yoga's purifying breath, maybe even it's colon cleanse. It's a quest to figure out how a practice rooted in renunciation and aimed at enlightenment has become such a business behemoth. It's a journey that touches on purity, desire, freedom, vanity, hope, madness and, believe it or not, bioterrorism. It will mean peering into yoga's future, as well as looking back at its enigmatic past, the task we now turn ourselves to. So take a deep breath and let's begin.

1

Lights, Karma, Action!

Yoga is a mirror, to look at ourselves from within.
—B.K.S. IYENGAR, IYENGAR YOGA WEBSITE

Yoga is a phenomenon, an institution, an unstoppable cultural force that has embedded itself in just about every aspect of our lives. Pick up a magazine, go online or turn on the TV. There's yoga on the cover, yoga in the copy, and yoga in the ads. The coverage is almost uniformly upbeat, generating the kind of "positives" the average politician would kill for. Yoga, we are told, can help battle-scarred soldiers de-stress. It can ease the side effects of cancer treatment. It may even be able to prevent the onset of Alzheimer's.

So how did this obscure, esoteric Eastern discipline come to embody all the aspects deemed essential for living a healthy, satisfying and righteous modern life? Yoga's incredible malleability, its ability to reflect and refract the times, has something to do with it. Yoga can be all things to all people. To the workout junky, it's a "low-impact" health regimen. To the type-A stockbroker, it's all about stress relief and a shot at "centeredness." And to the spiritually inclined, yoga offers a path of small, slow steps toward enlightenment. It's West Coast and East Coast, Old School and New Style,

Alpha Male and Dominant Female. It's the energy that can unite our increasingly Balkanized world.

It wasn't always this way. The popular perception of yoga has changed immensely over time. Fledgling yoga was narrowly defined. It was the domain of only the drippy, its practitioners the target of endless ridicule. In later narratives, the yoga scene was a dark and seamy netherworld, an atmosphere shot through with promiscuity, fraud and lunacy. Eventually, yoga attained acceptance, then begrudging respect. Now yoga's status in our culture is almost unique: untouchable, untarnished, endlessly evolving, exempt from the vulgarity of overexposure and beyond the vicissitudes of fashion. This is the kind of brand awareness advertisers dream of at night.

Of course, this kind of cultural domination is bound to engender enemies, and yoga has them. For some people the whole yoga scene is, well, a crock. They see yoga as nothing more than watered-down mysticism or an overplayed fitness product, doled out in manageable sixty-minute servings by slick, marketable gurus. Anyway, what we do isn't really yoga, they say. But ask them to *define* yoga and all you'll get is a blank stare.

So what *is* yoga? The word *yoga* comes from the Sanskrit root *yuj*, which is most often translated to mean "union." That's reflected in the dictionary definition of yoga (depending on whose dictionary), which goes something like "a group of ancient mental and physical practices that develop self-awareness in order to create union between mind, body and spirit, leading to liberation." Ask the purists to define yoga and the answers will be along these lines. "The purpose of yoga is the development of self-awareness to the point of liberation," says Trisha Lamb, former head of the California-based Yoga Research and Education Center.[1] "Yoga is a method to attain enlightenment," says Sharon Gannon, head of the Jivamukti yoga studio in downtown New York.[2]

These definitions may come as a rude shock to those who think of yoga as a fast way to get smokin' abs, a firm butt or an elastic spine. But Hatha yoga, the physical poses practiced by most westerners, and by extension most people throughout the world, is just a razor-thin slice of the entire discipline. "Flexibility may be the secondary outcome of the practice of yoga, but it is not the purpose," says Yogi Amrit Desai, who oversees the Amrit Yoga Institute in Florida and who previously founded the Kripalu Center for Yoga and Health, arguably the largest and most established yoga retreat in North America. "There are many flexible miserable people in this world. So why be flexible and be miserable? Why not eliminate the misery? That's what the word *yoga* represents, how to eliminate all the misery," Desai says.[3]

James Barkan, owner of the Barkan Method teacher-training facility, agrees that yoga is first and foremost a *mental* discipline. "It's not about contorting your body in all kinds of weird positions. Yoga is about quieting the mind so that you can connect to it," he says.[4] Baron Baptiste, founder of the Baptiste Power Vinyasa yoga technique, agrees. "The technical knowledge, that just helps us protect our knees, our spine, our necks, so it's safe and it helps us be more effective in the physical yoga practice," he says. "Really, it's the mind, the techniques of opening and focusing the mind."[5] Yoga teacher and competitor Tony Sanchez, director and founder of the Academia de Yoga in San Jose del Cabo, Mexico, says, "My definition of yoga is concentration.... Having the concentration will allow you to reach deeper and deeper into your own self. Therefore you will have a lot more understanding of who you are and what your main purpose is to be."[6]

It gets more complicated when you consider the mind-boggling array of yoga styles that have been developed over the years by various gurus, all springing from different lineages and traditions, each of them requiring its own definition, or at least its own branding. Amrit Desai calls his Amrit Method "meditation in motion," an approach that "integrates joyful inner stillness with effortless outer action." Baron Baptiste calls his Baptiste Power Vinyasa yoga "a dynamic combination of strength, sweat and spirituality." Anusara yoga creator John Friend says his yoga system "unifies a Tantric philosophy of intrinsic Goodness with Universal Principles of Alignment."

Now, don't be surprised if some of this sounds vaguely ... religious. Yoga is closely connected to the dharmic faiths of Hinduism, Buddhism, Jainism and Sikhism. But yoga itself is not a religion.

Yoga has no deity to worship, no services to attend, no sacred icons, no formal creed, no ordained clergy or priests and no system of temples or churches. In fact, the relationship between yoga and religion is often an uneasy one, especially in the modern, Western context. "Yoga is without religion. Yoga is without tradition. Tradition, religion, this type of thing is man-made," says Baron Baptiste. "I don't need something from the outside telling me how to live. Religion is for that purpose." Buddhist practitioner Trisha Lamb agrees yoga is not religion but is quick to point out that it "can help anybody's religious practice because of the calmness and centeredness that it gives you." Journalist and yogini Elizabeth Kadetsky notes, "You hear a lot of people today saying, 'Yoga is for everyone, yoga is a universal religion.' "[7] Yet many people are attracted to yoga precisely because it lacks the rigidity of established religions. So yoga has it both ways—appealing to people looking for a spiritual experience, but not so dogmatic as to scare anyone off.

Adding to yoga's appeal is that there is still some mystery to it. "We like this mystical side, that there's just this one quality or X factor that we can't answer," Kadetsky says. This inexplicable quality also plays into Western ideas about the mysterious East, the far-off and magical Orient. "The East has always provided a blank screen," Kadetsky says. And through yoga we can "imagine a perfect system of what we want that our own traditions don't give us."

In the Beginning

There is a downside to all this ambiguity. It makes separating yoga fact from yoga fiction a Sisyphean task. Let's start with what we do know. Yoga began somewhere in India. Well, what was, back then, the Indus Valley region, land that's now home to western India and modern-day Pakistan. Around four thousand years ago, this area was the seat of the Indus Valley civilization, also known as the Harrapan. Archaeologists have been unearthing remains of Harrapan life since 1922, when the first clues to this previously undiscovered society were revealed. Evidence suggests that Indus Valley cities were efficient, well-ordered affairs, with straight streets, two-story baked-brick homes and rudimentary clay plumbing. And among all the petrified goodies archaeologists have unearthed (ornamental

Growth Industry

Select results of the 2008 Yoga in America market study, commissioned by *Yoga Journal* and collected by the Harris Interactive Service Bureau:

- Americans spend US$5.7 billion a year on yoga classes and products, including equipment, clothing, vacations and media (DVDs, videos, books and magazines). This figure represents an increase of 87% compared with the previous study in 2004.
- Almost 7 percent of American adults, or 15.8 million people practice yoga, down slightly from the 2004 figure of 16.5 million. Of the yoga practitioners surveyed:
  - 72.2% are women; 27.8% are men
  - 40.6% are 18 to 34 years old; 41% are 35 to 54; and 18.4% are over 55
  - 71.4% are college educated; 27% have postgraduate degrees
  - 44% of yogis have yearly household incomes of US$75,000 or more; 24% have incomes of more than US$100,000

Results from a 2005 survey conducted by Canada's Print Measure Bureau show that

- 5.5% of Canadian adults, or 1.4 million people, now practice yoga, an increase of 15% from the prior year and 45.4% from 2003
- The fastest-growing segment is the 18 to 34 age group, which increased by 25.7% in one year
- About 2.1 million Canadians, or 1 in 12 non-practitioners, say they intend to try yoga within the next 12 months

Of the Canadian practitioners surveyed

- 72.3% are women, 27.7% are men
- 44.7% are 18 to 34 years old; 41% are 35 to 54

bracelets, the obligatory pots) was something of particular interest to yoga scholars—a stone seal depicting a nude male deity seated in what looks like a yogic meditation posture. Okay, it's not much. It's hardly definitive archaeological evidence of how to do a proper eagle pose, but it's a start. It tells us that sometime way back, somebody important was doing something that looked like yoga.

Textual evidence of yoga doesn't appear until many years later. The word *yoga* first surfaces around 1500 B.C., in four Brahmin scriptures known as the Vedas. The oldest, Rig Veda, a collection of hymns or mantras, defines yoga as "yoking" or "discipline." Another mention in the Atharva Veda refers to pranayama, a type of breath control that remains a central concept of yoga practice today. Yoga plays a more prominent role in the Upanishads, the sacred texts of ancient Hinduism that date from somewhere between 800 and 500 B.C. In these texts, yoga is generally and broadly defined as a discipline used to achieve liberation from suffering. The Upanishads also outline other concepts relevant to some versions of present-day yoga, such as universal consciousness, reincarnation and karma. The Upanishads contain specific instructions for binding the breath and the mind using the syllable *om*. The first mantra! Now we're getting somewhere. The epic Sanskrit text the Bhagavad Gita ("The Lord's Song"), which grew out of the literature of the Upanishads and was written some time between 500 and 100 B.C., elaborates further on yoga, outlining a threefold yogic path: Karma yoga, the path of service, and Jnana yoga, the path of wisdom or knowledge, together with Bhakti yoga, the path of devotion.

The first systematic presentation of yoga—and the one ancient yogic text that most of today's yoga teachers can claim some familiarity with—is the Yoga Sutras, 195 aphorisms probably compiled sometime between 300 and 100 B.C. by a sage named Patanjali. (The next time you hear yogis talking about the "two-thousand-year-old yoga tradition," you'll know it's Patanjali and his Yoga Sutras that they're most likely referring to.) Today Patanjali is widely regarded as the father of modern yoga, revered for codifying this ancient, oral tradition into what has become a practical blueprint for daily living. However, there's precious little evidence about who or even *what* Patanjali actually was. "There is a lot of mythology about Patanjali," says Kadetsky, including the theory that "he was a worm that dropped down from a tree and fell into the hands of a woman and was born as the god Patanjali."

Worm, man or god, Patanjali sure knew his yoga. In the Yoga Sutras he wrote that only hard work (Karma yoga) and deep meditation (Jnana yoga) could bring relief from suffering and lead to liberation. In addition, Patanjali believed humans suffered when they became attached to external phenomena and pulled away from their connection to a higher consciousness. The answer, he postulated, was Raja yoga, a system for control of the mind. Patanjali defined the word *yoga* as *Yoga citta vritti nirodha,* which basically means "Yoga is the restriction of the fluctuations of the conscious mind." Patanjali believed the conscious mind actively seeks experience outside itself, regardless of whether that experience is pleasurable or painful. Only cessation *(nirodha)* of these fluctuations *(vritti)* brings true liberation.

Patanjali's greatest legacy and the innovation that has elevated him into the pantheon of yoga royalty was the introduction of his "eight-limbed path" of yoga, or Ashtanga yoga. (Of course, Patanjali's Ashtanga yoga is not to be confused with Ashtanga-*style* yoga, a distinct, modern and copyrighted yoga method.) Patanjali's Ashtanga yoga progresses through these eight limbs, beginning with purification of the mind and spirit and coming to the body through postures (*asanas*) and breath control. This prepared the yogi for the subsequent stages of concentration and meditation. The process ends, eventually, with *samadhi,* liberation. It's rigorous stuff, nothing you could cram in on your lunch break or after work one day.

The next most important Hatha yoga text comes possibly as late as the eighteenth century. The Shiva Samhita describes eighty-four asanas, many of which had never been recorded before. According to the Shiva Samhita, and like all Hatha yoga philosophy of the time, the aim of performing asanas was to cure disease and bestow upon the yogi magical powers. (Shame that's gone by the wayside.) Among the Shiva Samhita's more radical declarations was the belief that even common householders could practice and benefit from yoga. (As long as they were male, of course; before the twentieth century, women doing Hatha yoga was practically unheard of.)

Notice, too, that asana is only one of Patanjali's eight limbs. Even for the "father of yoga," the physical poses were merely an early and intermediate step toward liberation. Hatha yoga, the purely physical regimen based on the yoga asanas, didn't develop as a separate practice until probably the ninth or tenth century B.C. The first texts devoted exclusively to Hatha yoga are more than likely treatises written by the guru Goraksha (or Gorakshanatha or Gorknath) during this period. Fast-forward a few centuries, to sometime during the mid-fourteenth century, and we meet Goraksha's disciple Svatmarama Yogin, who wrote the quintessential Hatha yoga treatise, the Hatha Yoga Pradipika. It's a slim discourse, however, describing just sixteen postures, and most of those variations on just one posture, the cross-legged lotus pose familiar to yogis and non-yogis alike.

The Hatha yoga of old has little resemblance to today's sweaty, souped-up workouts. Ancient yogis performed intense purification rituals before they would even begin the poses. Most present-day yogis spend five minutes doing breathing exercises that they're happy to have out of the way. The ancient yogis hoped to gain enlightenment by transforming their physical bodies into divine vessels impervious to disease and devoid of any defects. Present-day yogis want to look good naked. Ancient yogis had to master the intricate physiology of the human body by learning about the muscles, organs and tissue. Present-day yogis want to learn about the muscles, organs and tissue of that slinky yogini doing the scorpion pose next to them.

2

Cowboys and Indians

This, the firm holding back of the senses, is what is
called Yoga. He must be free from thoughtlessness
then, for Yoga comes and goes.
—KATHA UPANISHAD, 6.11, *THE UPANISHADS, PART II*

Yoga may have begun its long march west as far back as 1784, a century before official British colonial rule of India began, when Sir William Jones founded the Asiatic Society in Kolkata (then known as Calcutta). Aimed at enhancing and furthering the cause of Oriental research, the society undertook essays on the Vedas and yoga and compiled the first English-language translations of the Bhagavad Gita and Upanishads. But this was heady, academic stuff. The fun didn't really begin until the nineteenth century, when many westerners became seduced by Hatha yoga, which they saw as an out-of-body shortcut, a way to transcend the physical realm. Germans in particular were fascinated by Hatha yoga and yoga philosophy. From the 1830s through the rest of the century, many yoga texts were translated into German. The highlight was a German version of Svatmarama's Hatha Yoga Pradipika that came with beautiful but completely inaccurate watercolor illustrations, based as they were on written descriptions. Nevertheless, the text was highly influential, helping to elevate Hatha yoga above all other forms of the discipline.

The yogic books were also being translated into Sanskrit during this period, making them widely available to the average Indian reader for the first time. New ideas about Indian nationalism and independence were also beginning to foment, and many Indians felt it was their duty to rediscover and reclaim yoga. "There were a lot of people who felt that the true ancient Indian tradition needed to be resurrected," Kadetsky explains, "so that Indians could have a better self-perception and more confidence and have the self-confidence to break away from the British."

An interest in all things Eastern was also taking hold across the seas, in the Americas. A group of influential American intellectuals, including Henry David Thoreau, Louisa May Alcott and Ralph Waldo Emerson (you didn't *have* to have three names), had taken to calling themselves the Transcendentalists. In rejecting the trappings of nineteenth-century American society, the Transcendentalists gave birth to new ideas about literature, culture and, especially, religion. They believed in an ideal spiritual state that transcended the physical and that could be realized only through the individual's intuition, rather than religious doctrine. The group drew much of its inspiration from Vedic scripture and the Bhagavad Gita. "I owed a magnificent day to the Bhagavat-Gita. It was the first of books; it was as if an empire spake to us," Emerson wrote in his diary on October 1, 1848.[1]

"The biggest misconception [about yoga] is that it really became popular or practiced or known in a significant way in the United States in the sixties. You have to back that up by about a century," says author Stefanie Syman, who studied the Transcendentalists' influence on yoga culture for a book she's writing called *Practice: A History of Yoga in America*. "It wasn't that the Transcendentalists or people in the nineteenth century were practicing yoga, but there was definitely a growing awareness and definitely a deep interest in Hinduism and Eastern philosophies," she says.[2]

Jump forward thirty years and a Russian immigrant improbably named Madame Blavatsky was captivating New York City audiences with lectures that explored the secrets of the ancient Vedas. In 1875 Blavatsky had established the Theosophical Society, ostensibly a religious order. It was a theological hodgepodge, a smattering of

Hinduism, a sprinkling of Buddhism, stirred up with some home-grown ideas closely resembling reincarnation and karma. The proclivities of some society members, including Blavatsky, ran closer to the occult, and their accounts of clairvoyance and levitation naturally made them media darlings.

All this metaphysical action primed late-nineteenth-century westerners for what has come to be seen as a seminal event in yoga history. In 1893 a charismatic Hindu leader and philosopher named Swami Vivekananda became the first Indian spiritual teacher to speak publicly and passionately in North America about Hinduism, including the study of yoga and meditation. Vivekananda was an instant success when he addressed the first Parliament of the World's Religions during the Chicago World's Fair. Dubbed the "Cyclonic Monk" for his electric speaking style, he earned wild two-minute applause after delivering a renowned lecture beginning not with the familiar "Ladies and gentlemen" but with "Sisters and brothers of America," or so the legend goes.[3] The *Boston Evening Transcript* described him as "the most striking figure" at the parliament, adding that "years of voluntary poverty and homeless wanderings have not robbed him of his birthright of gentleman."[4]

"Other Indian teachers had come west and talked about the Bhagavad Gita and other ancient spiritual ideas with some success. But Vivekananda was the first to sit people down and teach them how to meditate," says Syman. "He was one of the first to start talking about yoga in scientific terms." Vivekananda's success catapulted him to fame, leading him to give lectures across America, teaching yoga and meditation in cities as far-flung as Memphis, San Francisco, New York, Los Angeles and St. Louis. In 1894 he set up the New York Vedanta Society, an organization dedicated to yoga and Vedic study. (Today there are over thirty Vedanta societies spread across the globe, from Toronto to Tel Aviv.) After four years of constant touring in the West, Vivekananda returned to India in 1897. He died five years later. A memorial plaque near the site where Vivekananda first addressed the crowds in Chicago states, "His unprecedented success opened the way for dialogue between Eastern and Western religions."

There's a bittersweet irony to Vivekananda's story. According to Syman, Vivekananda "did not come to America to teach yoga. He came to raise money. He wanted to help impoverished Indians, because he had seen how much they were suffering." As Vivekananda himself explained to one American questioner at the time, "I do not preach any religion. I have come here to earn something to help the poor in India." But the Cyclonic Monk had much better luck as a teacher than as a profiteer. The money he raised was "not nearly as much as he had hoped. It was only after being here for a while and talking to small groups of Americans that he began to preach more actively and see his role as a teacher of yoga," Syman explains. And in this employment he *was* successful, attracting a dedicated following of socialites, feminists and prodigal sons from families with names like Vanderbilt, Rutherford and Goodrich.

As a result of Vivekananda's success, and emboldened by the growing influence of groups such as Blavatsky's Theosophists, a stream of Eastern mystics and holy men began landing on turn-of-the-century American shores. Swamis became a kind of mascot, as the upper classes began "practicing" yoga in greater numbers, and increasingly as a complete way of life. "While people had been drawn to yoga for the physical asana practice, they understood it as a complete system. To just do the poses was not to do yoga at that time," says Syman, although some westerners had already begun bending yoga to their will, redefining it to fit their needs. "Even in the mid-nineteenth century, Thoreau was complaining that things were too loud," Syman says. As a result, yoga of the time was often promoted as "an anti-capitalist technique," Syman says. "Here was a way of counteracting the speed and intensity of American capitalism."

Hoodoo Gurus

The mainstream culture of the time viewed yoga as something below ridiculous, a kooky pursuit best left to overeducated elitist oddballs. But as yoga became more fashionable, controversy was almost inevitable. And when the backlash began, it was the newest Americans who found themselves embroiled in the mess. South Asians were about to become the new century's new bogeymen.

Over 20 million immigrants arrived into the United States in the forty years between 1870 and 1910. Xenophobia was on the rise, however, and San Francisco, now thought of as a beacon of broad-mindedness, was ground zero for turn-of-the-century intolerance. In May 1905 sixty-seven labor unions came together to form the Asiatic Exclusion League (AEL), its stated aim being to spread anti-Asian propaganda and influence legislation restricting Asian immigration. Three years later the AEL reported 231 affiliated organizations. In 1907 a sister organization with the same name was formed in Vancouver, with its own stated aim of keeping "Oriental immigrants out of British Columbia." The situation in Vancouver was even worse than that across the border. One night in September 1907, following a series of inflammatory racist speeches at Vancouver's City Hall, nearly nine thousand league members took to the streets, besieging the city's Asian neighborhoods, shouting racist slogans and causing thousands of dollars' worth of damage.

While the initial targets of both leagues were Japanese, Chinese and Korean immigrants, the scope soon widened beyond the "yellow peril," taking in all East Asians, including the ballooning number of Indian immigrants. With the American AEL's influential membership pressuring to enact new legislation, the chips soon fell. In 1906 the San Francisco Board of Education agreed to segregate Asian schoolchildren. And on February 5, 1917, Congress forcibly passed the sweeping and controversial Immigration Act of 1917 with an overwhelming majority, overriding President Woodrow Wilson's veto. The list of undesirables already banned from entering the United States included "idiots," "feeble-minded persons," "epileptics," "insane persons," alcoholics, professional beggars, all persons "mentally or physically defective," polygamists and anarchists. Congress then widened the restrictions by unceremoniously implementing an Asiatic Barred Zone. With the stroke of a pen, people from much of Asia and the Pacific islands could no longer immigrate to the United States. The act was not repealed until 1965.

All of this dovetailed nicely with the American spiritual reform movement, which saw its desperate task as trying to reorient (so to speak) America's wayward moral compass. In this atmosphere, any group with unpopular ideas and peopled by dark-skinned foreigners could find itself designated a cult. The media's take on all things South Asian shifted in lockstep. A particularly harsh spotlight was thrown on Indians, as anything even faintly "Hindoo" took on a sinister taint. There were calls to fight back against this "Turban Tide." The resulting depictions were curious and confused. A typical editorial cartoon of a malodorous lay-about "Hindu" shows him wearing the turban of Sikhism.[5] And so on.

As time wore on, yoga would be dragged into the scuffle, and often through its Western adepts. "There was still a lot of anti-Hindu sentiment and anti-cult sentiment. So yoga and the people teaching it were often meshed in that acrimony," says Syman. One mysterious figure in particular became the media's favorite Western whipping boy—although he brought much of the trouble on himself. Pierre Bernard was an American-born yogi, scholar, occultist, mystic and founder of no fewer than three influential spiritual groups: the Tantrik Order in America, the New York Sanskrit College and the Clarkstown Country Club. Bernard, who described himself as "a curious combination of the business man and the religious scholar," was the first American to carry Vivekananda's torch of yoga and Hinduism. But not without inflicting some severe damage on yoga's reputation.

Early facts surrounding Bernard's life are scarce. He was born Perry Baker (or Peter Coon, or Coons or possibly even Bernard) in 1875 in Leon, Iowa (or somewhere in the Midwest), to a family of lawyers and doctors. Or maybe they were barbers. Early in life he, too, worked as a barber around Illinois and California. Later years were reportedly spent traveling America, working itinerantly as a fruit picker, acrobat and salmon packer. By 1905, having returned from one of many trips to India, this man of mystery was now going by the name Pierre Arnold Bernard and calling himself a yogi. Bernard clearly was familiar with yogic philosophy, but made all sorts of wild claims regarding other aspects of his résumé, including claiming that he was a physician, according to Syman.

By 1906 Bernard had established the Tantrik Order in America. The group was dedicated in part to the study of the tantras, an aspect of Hindu scripture. However, the emphasis seemed to be on the more esoteric practices, full of magic, ritual and mysticism. In 1910 Bernard established his second religious order in New York, the New York Sanskrit College, also known, provocatively, as the Temple of Mystery. Offering courses in yoga, Sanskrit and religion, the college attracted some of the city's best and brightest. Around this time Bernard met and soon married a dancer, interior decorator and yoga teacher known by the equally exotic, equally unlikely but quite real name of Blanche DeVries.

Then it all went wrong. In 1910 a teenage follower of Bernard's named Zelda Hopp (where did they get these names?) told police that Bernard had taken her into a locked room at the college, ordered her to strip and put his hand on her left breast to test her heartbeat, part of her alleged induction into the order. Police raided the college headquarters and were perplexed by what they found: canvas-covered mattresses, an inner circle participating in secret rites, talk of blood oaths and secret handshakes. Neighbors told investigators even more salacious tales. "What my wife and I have seen through the windows of that place is scandalous. We saw men and women in various stages of deshabille. Women's screams mingled with wild Oriental music," neighbor F.H. Gans told police.[6]

Bernard was arrested and charged with kidnapping Hopp and another follower. The trial was a circus. The press had already given Bernard a new moniker, Oom the Omnipotent. (Why "Oom" is anyone's guess.) A typical headline trumpeted, "Omnipotent Oom, the Guru of the Loving Tantriks." There were daily accounts of "Oriental sanctums" and girls kidnapped to serve as sex slaves. "Police Break in on Weird Hindu Rites Girls and Men Mystics Cease Strange Dance as 'Priest' Is Arrested," screamed a headline from William Randolph Hearst's *New York American*.[7]

But the charges against "Oom" wouldn't stick. The victims refused to testify because, according to the press, Oom held such mental power over them that he could reduce them to tears on the stand, rendering them unable to testify. The girls' actions seemed to support this wild hypothesis. "Zelda is too ill to prosecute the great Oom," a family spokesman claimed. With the case dismissed, Bernard was free to go back to business—although with a soiled reputation and a new name he hated and could never shake.

According to Robert Love's excellent online article "Fear of Yoga," about the changing depiction of the discipline, cases like Oom's whetted the growing Western appetite for stories that intermingled yoga with squalor, sex, insanity and slavery. It was the oldest trick in the headline writer's book, and it worked. Love cites a 1911 *Los Angeles Times* story headlined "A Hindu Apple for Modern Eve: The Cult of the Yogis Lures Women to Destruction." The point of the article was unclear, but it didn't matter. The mention of "dusky-hued Orientals" who sat on "drawing-room sofas, the center of admiring attention, while fair hands passed them cakes and served them tea" was enough to entice readers. *Current Literature* also weighed in with a 1911 article titled "The Heathen Invasion of America," postulating that yoga "leads to domestic infelicity, and insanity and death." (Other spicy headlines uncovered by Love include "Rich Worship Love Goddess Along Riviera," "Orgies of Super-Love Cult Send Five to Jail" and "High School Girls on Grill.")[8]

The drumbeat had now reached the halls of power. "Agents are now quietly at work, investigating the strange spread of these Oriental religions throughout this country," *The Washington Post* reported in 1912. The article told the world about Miss Sarah Farnum, who "gave her entire fortune" for a Hindu summer school, and Miss Aloise Reuss, who was sent to the Illinois Insane Asylum, and Mrs. May Wright Sewell, who was made "dangerously ill" by the teachings of her yogi.[9]

By 1919, perhaps to escape all this, Pierre Bernard moved operations out of New York City to an estate thirty miles north that he'd acquired as a gift from a disciple who'd been an Episcopalian nun. There Bernard set up something he called the Braeburn Country Club. Passersby the club, it was said, would be treated to the sight of a hundred Braeburn-ites exercising, all dressed alike in bloomers and sandals. "You could call it the first American ashram, but it was in some ways much more of a country club that was founded on yoga principles," says Syman.

Bernard eventually established another proto-ashram he called the Clarkstown Country Club (CCC). It became one of the most influential organizations in the development of Western yoga—and along the way allowed Bernard to reclaim his tarnished reputation.

The CCC was an empire of intellectualism, with a famed library that attracted scholars and researchers from around the world, who came to feast on Bernard's exalted collection of esoterica and exotica. The CCC was imperial in scope, too. There were six tennis courts, indoor and outdoor swimming pools, elaborate gardens, a miniature zoo, a cabin cruiser moored on the Hudson River, a sports stadium with night lighting, a theater, two gymnasiums, billiard and cards rooms, a playroom for children, artist studios and a powerful rooftop telescope. The CCC also operated a circus, under the largest privately owned tent in the United States. The highlight was a performance by nine elephants, all of them acquired and trained by Bernard. (It was the elephants that somehow powered the night lighting and PA system for the sports stadium.)

By the late thirties, Bernard was just another affluent riverfront country-club manager. By the time of his death in 1955, Pierre Bernard was also a bank president, an officer on the Nyack chamber of commerce and a member of more than twenty societies, including the Royal Society of Arts, the Royal Asiatic Society and the Freemasons. But it didn't matter how respectable yogis like Bernard came to be. The damage to yoga had been done.

It would take another good old-fashioned Indian guru to begin to set things straight. He came in the form of Mukunda Lal Ghosh, who'd become better known as Yogananda. Born into a devout Bengali family in Gorakhpur, India, Yogananda was a mystical wunderkind, said to have an awareness of spirituality far beyond his tender years. In 1910, at the age of just twenty-four, he founded the Yogoda Satsanga Society of India, a school that combined education, yoga and philosophy. That school was the first building block of what would become a vast spiritual organization. Its headquarters would be far away, however, in a land called America.

Yogananda first came to the United States in 1920 to attend the International Congress of Religious Liberals in Boston. Within the year Yogananda had founded the Self-Realization Fellowship, an organization devoted to disseminating his teachings on yoga, meditation and the nature of God. This was a more rigorous and haughty yoga than most westerners had yet tangled with, even those familiar

---

Hindoo Headliners

A piecemeal journey through the archives of the *Los Angeles Times.*

"Judge Scalps Hindu; Makes East Indian Doff His Bright Yellow Turban in Court—Pate Bald as Marble"
February 17, 1914

"Back in Good Graces: Another Queer Chapter Written in the Love Affair of Founder of East Indian Cult"
April 2, 1914

"Swami Buys Swanky Automobile"
December 6, 1925

"Ardent Love Making Laid to Asserted Fake Hindu"
May 1, 1930

"Witness Swears by Allah He Can't Tell Marihuana"
November 18, 1931

"Did Hindu Do Such a Deed?"
December 1, 1931

"News of the San Joaquin Valley; Hindu Murder Ring Quiz Begun"
June 14, 1933

---

with Pierre Bernard's heady sermons. Like his Western counterparts, Yogananda was not above a little self-promotion. According to Syman, he had "a well-oiled machine for promoting his yoga, which included mail order courses and a thriving organization in Los Angeles." Los Angeles soon became the official international headquarters for his fellowship.

The fellowship was a well-regarded institution and Yogananda a highly sought after mystical figure. Among his students were many prominent figures in science, business and the arts, including horticulturist Luther Burbank; George Eastman, inventor of the Kodak camera; and poet Edwin Markham. Yogananda was even received at the White House in 1927 by President Calvin Coolidge, who'd become interested in his spiritual exploits.

To the tabloids, however, Yogananda was just another target in a turban. Newspaper headlines proclaimed him "Swami Yogananda, East Indian Love Cult Leader."[10] Reporters recounted in detail his run-in with Los Angeles police over property-fraud charges. It was clear the anti-Asian and anti-Hindu hysteria that had gripped the nation twenty years earlier had not subsided. In fact, a movement was afoot to formalize it. The Immigration Act of 1917 that had prohibited immigration from the Asiatic Barred Zone also imposed a literacy test on new immigrants. When the literacy test alone failed to prevent most potential immigrants from entering the United States, members of Congress sought a new way to restrict immigration, enacting them as law with the passing of the Immigration Act of 1924 (the Johnson-Reed Act). Existing nationality laws from 1790 and 1870 already excluded people of Asian lineage from becoming naturalized. Further provisions in the new act prohibited any alien from immigrating who by virtue of race or nationality was ineligible for citizenship—thereby ensuring that all Asians, including Indians, would no longer be admitted to the United States. For those Indians already here, such as Yogananda, tolerance was an uphill battle. Forget acceptance.

Despite what mainstream America thought of him, it was Yogananda who had the last laugh. In 1946 Yogananda published his life story, *Autobiography of a Yogi,* six years before his death at the age of fifty-nine. More than a decade later, during the civil and social paroxysms of the sixties, the book became a virtual bible of the counterculture. It has since been translated into eighteen languages and remains a bestseller to this day. It was not the only way Yogananda would flourish in death. After he was interred at the Forest Lawn Memorial Park in Los Angeles (alongside the likes of

Clark Gable, Carole Lombard, Jimmy Stewart and Humphrey Bogart), Yogananda's obituary in *Time* magazine quoted excerpts from a letter written by the mortuary's director: "No physical disintegration was visible.… Even 20 days after death … Paramahansa Yogananda's body was apparently devoid of impurities.… [His] case is unique in our experience."[11]

The Long Road Back

Yoga would get back into the culture's good graces not through its lure of mental clarity but for its promise of a more perfect earthly frame. And it would be aided immensely by the work of the famed guru Krishnamacharya. The rigorously physical mode of Hatha yoga he pioneered soon found favor in the West and is the basis for many of today's brawny yoga styles.

Accepting the legend of Krishnamacharya requires a fairly hefty suspension of disbelief. Unfolding in ancient caves, peopled by wild-eyed mystics, the narrative is improbable and scattershot, built on myth, mystery and plain old make-believe. Krishnamacharya's beginnings were simple enough. Born in 1888 in the southwestern India city of Chitradurga, Krishnamacharya was just five years old when his father began teaching him Patanjali's Yoga Sutras. He continued to hone his yogic skills during his years of study, often being asked to school others.

From here it gets wacky. At age twelve, Krishnamacharya claimed to have received the ancient teachings of a long-lost yogic text during a dream. In years to come, subsequent visions would lead him to an ancient cave in Tibet, where he discovered a 230-year-old hermit. For seven years the hermit schooled him in the secret techniques of yoga. The hermit then told his apprentice to do something that had never been done before—bring this newly discovered yoga lineage to the masses. Some yoga converts take the Krishnamacharya story as gospel; others don't buy a word of it. It doesn't much matter either way. The point is that the genie was now out of the bottle. "There was a zeitgeist that suddenly this tradition, that either didn't exist and was being invented, or that did exist but only in extreme secrecy, should be disseminated to the public," says journalist and yogini Elizabeth Kadetsky. "As the official Indian version of the yoga story goes, this was what brought this two-thousand-year unbroken tradition into the public."

And disseminate Krishnamacharya did. In 1924 he crossed paths with the maharaja of Mysore, a great yoga enthusiast. At the turn of the nineteenth century, the Mysore royal family had hired a British gymnast to teach the young princes gymnastics. Now that the maharaja's tastes ran toward the homegrown and esoteric, he decided to open a yoga school. Krishnamacharya would be its teacher.

The key to Krishnamacharya's success was his ability to innovate. He'd often tailor his teachings to suit the crowd. His buff bourgeois students weren't much interested in the supernatural dimensions of the practice. (Sound familiar?) They were interested in building strength and fitness. With access to the former gymnasium's manual and aids, such as wall ropes and blocks, Krishnamacharya soon found himself incorporating the equipment into his yoga routines. These yoga props are still used within this yoga lineage today.

Among Krishnamacharya's protégés were B.K.S. Iyengar and Pattabhi Jois, two legendary yoga figures still active on the circuit. The maharaja paid for Krishnamacharya and his two acolytes to take their show on the road, and the three of them brought yoga demonstrations to appreciative and diverse audiences across India, fueling a revival in this homegrown art. These glory days ended quickly, however. After the nation won independence from England, the new Indian political establishment promptly dethroned the maharaja, and Krishnamacharya said goodbye to his sugar daddy. He moved to Bangalore, then to Chennai, where he lived and taught until he slipped into a coma and died, in 1989, at 101 years of age.

Back home yoga was getting mixed up with that most American of concoctions, the cult of celebrity. During the thirties, gossip columnists such as Louella Parsons and Leonard Lyons were coming into their own. They saw their work as ordaining the new high priests and priestesses of the fame cult, and filled endless column inches with the gallivanting and goings-on of the Hollywood set—which now included yoga. These stargazers outed a long list of yogis, according to Robert Love's supremely well-researched article "Fear of Yoga"; Cole Porter was using yoga to recover from a riding accident, Greta Garbo liked to practice alone, and even Mae West was mad for yoga.[12]

The media's approach to yoga had softened. The tone had become tolerant, even charitable. Yoga's sinister edge was a thing of the past. Nobody, it seemed, could be much bothered with dredging up yoga's dark side anymore, not since Maureen O'Sullivan, Robert Ryan and even Joan Crawford had taken it up. Even the infamous English occultist, hedonist, drug experimenter and social critic Aleister Crowley, once dubbed "The Wickedest Man in the World" by quarters of the English press, could publish a 1939 book called *Eight Lectures on Yoga* without a fuss. (Crowley's aim was simple, as he took great pains to point out in the book. He merely wanted to "explain the subject of Yoga in clear language" because "like all great things, it is masked by confused thinking; and, only too often, brought into contempt by the machinations of knavery.")[13]

The person who benefited most from yoga's rediscovered respectability was a petite young woman named Indra Devi, who came to be known as the "First Lady of Yoga." Devi's life spanned three centuries. She was born Eugenie Peterson in May 1899 in tsarist Russia, and her formative years came during the Bolshevik Revolution. Once the Communists were in power, Peterson and her mother left Russia. After traveling across Europe as an actress and dancer, Peterson relocated to India in 1927, attracted by the country's culture and religiosity. She continued to act, now under the stage name Indra Devi. But she also wanted to study yoga and so set her sights on the brilliant but mercurial Krishnamacharya. Becoming the first Western woman to study with Krishnamacharya would not be easy. "There's a famous story that he refused to teach her at first. She persisted, *and* she got the maharaja of Mysore to pull some strings," says Syman. "And finally Krishnamacharya relented."

Krishnamacharya was evidently pleased with his disciple, urging her to go out and teach yoga throughout India, a first for a Western woman. When Devi and her husband moved to China, she opened what was surely China's first yoga school, in the house of Madame Chiang Kai-shek, wife of the nationalist Chinese leader. Devi returned to India after World War Two. After her husband died,

Devi was on the move again, this time heading west. "She comes to America, opens a studio on Sunset Boulevard and starts teaching starlets," Syman recounts. Today she is best remembered for giving this misunderstood Indian tradition a female, European face. And a famous face at that. Makeup guru Elizabeth Arden was an early advocate. Gloria Swanson became one of her best friends. It "made an average man think that there must be something to Yoga after all, if it has been taken up by so many prominent personalities," Devi told the World Vegetarian Congress in 1957."[14]

Devi's first book, *Forever Young Forever Healthy,* marketed her practice as a technique for achieving vitality. "Yoga is an art and science of living," she was fond of saying.[15] Notice, however, that the word *yoga* is not in the book's title. Devi wanted the emphasis on lifestyle, not on mysticism. "She was the first to succeed in presenting yoga in a mass way. And the way she did that was by further pulling it apart from Hinduism," Syman contends. "[These were] the postwar years and America was a somewhat conservative place. We were not interested in the mystical aspects of culture ... Indra Devi was accommodating the national temper."

In 1953 Indra Devi married Los Angeles doctor and humanitarian Sigfrid Knauer. Fluent in five languages, Devi traveled tirelessly around the world giving conferences, eventually settling in Argentina after Knauer died in 1984, though she continued to travel around the world spreading her message of yoga and enlightenment for the next fifteen years. She died in 2002. She'd reached the ripe old age of 103.

Befitting the times, the fifties were a comparatively grandfatherly period for yoga. Much of the snap and zest had gone out of it as a media subject. The news that violinist and conductor Yehudi Menuhin was studying yoga with B.K.S. Iyengar was met with a shrug. And it was quietly noted that in 1955 bodybuilder Walt Baptiste, a former Mr. America, and his wife, Magana, had opened the first yoga studio on the West Coast, called the Center for Yoga and Health.

One yogi's career was getting off the ground during the fifties. After studying in India, Richard Hittleman returned to New York, his hometown, and began teaching yoga. Later he would publish a series of books, including *Yoga for Health* and *Yoga: 28 Day Exercise Plan,* simple treatises that continue to be popular today. Hittleman, who came from a conservative Jewish family, was a traditional yogi and thus bent on enlightenment. But he knew his audience and so presented instead a streamlined, secular practice. As his books sold millions, Hittleman began hanging tough with Beat-era big names such as Alan Watts and Jack Kerouac. He was also working out the details of a TV deal. A few years later that TV show would transform yoga.

As the sixties loomed, the culture at large had decided that enough danger and discomfort had been drained from yoga for it to become widely accepted. How bad could it be, now that Marilyn Monroe and Gary Cooper were on board? Yoga was here to stay. Now it was time for the Approved History of Yoga to begin. And for the money to really start rolling in.

3

Posers

Yoga in Mayfair or Fifth Avenue, or in any other
place which is on the telephone, is a spiritual fake.
—CARL JUNG, FROM *THE COLLECTED WORKS OF
C.G. JUNG*

Established religions, spiritual philosophies and self-improvement systems are growing in popularity worldwide. It's often hypothesized that this new zealotry springs from some deformity in the modern soul. We live too much in the Here and Wow. Too many decades of convenience, consumerism and carelessness have degraded our essence and made us metaphysically flabby, so the theory goes. As a result, many of us are searching for something solid, something ancient and unchanging, something that will satisfy our yearning for roots in an increasingly rootless world.

When these aspirants finally find what they've been looking for, they often embrace it tightly. It's the zeal of the new convert, a kind of excited apprehension about verifying and validating everything they've just learned. New converts also make the best evangelists. The same is true in yoga, despite that the practice has no tradition of proselytizing. In fact, both Hinduism and Buddhism, the two religions most aligned with yoga, generally reject conversion as an act of aggression. Yet it's always that friend who's just found yoga himself who's so desperate to drag you along. (The Enthusiastic

Period is usually limited, however. Invariably, the yoga missionary exhausts his or her passion for conversion, wears out the patience and heightens the immunity of close friends or ceases to have friends who haven't already been converted.)

Among the newer and perhaps more superficial Western yogis, this fledgling fundamentalism will often involve a two-week yoga "intensive" somewhere in India. Understandably eager for Western dollars, owners of the local yoga school, restaurant and hotel will try to ease their guests' transition to Indian life by mimicking as best they can how things might be back home. Thus westerners are assured an entirely inauthentic experience inside a hermetic bubble. It's a kind of Disneyland for yoga dilettantes, far removed from the daily grind. Without having any contact with actual Indians except their gurus and waiters, the pilgrims come away satisfied, even transformed. They've just gotten a taste of the "real yoga," after all. (These are often the same yogis who will later categorically state without corroboration or irony that modern yoga is nothing but a spectacle, an untenable corruption of the real thing.)

Any serious yoga scholar knows searching for the "real yoga" is folly, chiefly because of the inconvenient fact that no such thing ever existed. As we've seen, there's simply no evidence of a monolithic yoga tradition tracing back to an original, pristine source. Accepting the infallibility and antiquity of yogic teaching is a leap of faith.

The only thing more fruitless than trying to find the karmic well from which yoga sprang is trying to identify the moment when yoga veered "off course." Yoga fundamentalists, particularly the newly minted ones, tend to spend a lot of time looking for the tipping point, the instant or event that took yoga from esoteric purity to soulless enormity, as if it were possible to go back in time and correct it all. But if yoga's hazy history teaches us anything it's that there was no such tipping point. Yoga has always been veering off course.

There are two things about yoga's recent history we can say with certainty. The first is that the last four decades, what we might call the modern period of yoga, have brought enormous and, some might argue, cataclysmic changes. Yoga has gone through three major shifts in perception in that time alone. From the early sixties until the mid-seventies, yoga was seen as a nontoxic, drug-free high (the drug-fueled part came slightly later). From the late seventies to the late eighties, yoga was perceived as a yuppie pursuit, a New Age adjunct to the stress-relief and detox movements. And in the early nineties, yoga merged with the maturing fitness scene to birth the athleticization of yoga. Of course, these strands also overlapped and mingled together—resulting in today's complex and still-evolving yoga, a mash-up of everything that's come before.

The second is that plenty of gurus, seekers and savvy business folk have come along for the ride. What they've all been looking for is anyone's guess.

Instant Karma

If you can remember the sixties, the saying goes, you probably weren't there. A related paradox was true of yoga at that time: Whatever you could remember of yoga *before* the sixties you could now promptly forget. Even for the yogis who did live and breathe through those earlier decades, it seemed somehow that yoga didn't really "happen" until the sixties, when it was first catapulted into the upper echelons of popular culture—where it has remained firmly lodged ever since.

Of course, what happened during the sixties was merely the blooming of yogic ideas and innovations that had been maturing for decades. The real difference was that the media and culture at large had finally caught up. The times they were a-changin'. The flower-power generation welcomed yoga as a counterculture escape, a way to drop out while staying tuned in, says Stefanie Syman, author of the book *Practice: A History of Yoga in America*: "When the counterculture starts happening, people see this yoga thing and they see that when you turn it a little there's this whole dimension that really fits in with our whole idea of challenging Western materialism and rationalism and all the sacred cows of bourgeois middle-class society."

By the mid-sixties, *The New York Times* estimated that American yoga practitioners numbered between 20,000 and 100,000. Yet yogis still dwelt on the far fringes of society. "There was a big divide between people in middle America and people doing things that were 'alternative' at that point," says Trisha Lamb, former head of the Yoga Research and Education Center. "When I was a child," says Baron Baptiste, "people really didn't understand yoga. Even in San Francisco it was considered to be an oddity, a weird thing. You had to be a hippie or freak at some level to participate." The son of a yoga teacher, Baptiste recalls that "in school I was often referred to as Hare Krishna. I was teased a lot."

His father, Walt, had opened the Center for Yoga and Health in San Francisco in 1955, before Baron was born. In those days the average Joe stuck to the gym and steered pretty clear of the $5-per-month yoga classes. By the early sixties things were different. Yoga classes were filling up all over the United States, and the Center for Yoga and Health suddenly had new credibility. Thousands of students, socialites and celebrities (Lenny Bruce was one) visited the center over the next four decades, while the Baptiste family regularly hosted gurus from all over the world. "Very often they would stay in my parents' home," Baron says. The center also motivated Baron's choice of career. He learned to teach on the job by substituting for his father. In a 1996 article, *Yoga Journal* declared: "If there were a royal family of American yoga, Baron Baptiste would certainly be the prince."[1]

While Richard Hittleman's work in the fifties as a yoga instructor and author garnered him a loyal following, it was the sixties that made his a household name. In 1961 his *Yoga for Health* TV show began airing daily in Los Angeles, and by 1966 in New York as well. Many yogis consider the show to be the grandfather of today's booming instructional yoga business. (DVD copies of Hittleman's show are still in circulation.) Also in 1961, Yogananda's posthumous *Autobiography of a Yogi* became a sudden hit, what Syman calls "a must read for the time." Jockeying for top of the bestseller list was the very-much-alive Swami Vishnu-devananda, whose 1959 *Complete Illustrated Book of Yoga* had become another of the many essential mystical guidebooks. Vishnu-devananda's extensive travels throughout North America earned him the nickname "The Flying Guru." He eventually landed in Montreal and opened a spiritual retreat called the Sivananda Yoga Vedanta Centre. It's now one of the largest networks of yoga schools in the world, claiming ashrams in Asia, North and South America, the Caribbean and throughout Europe.

Nineteen sixty-five was a watershed year for North American yoga. In the United States the 1924 quota on Indian immigration to the United States was finally lifted. In Canada similarly tight restrictions on South Asian immigration were also revoked. The doors to the West were once again open. Within months you couldn't cross the street without bumping into a guru or discovering a new spiritual order. While some of these gallivanting Godmen came and went without a trace, many more found a toehold, and continue to influence the culture today.

Although Amrit Desai came to the United States in 1960 to study design, his true love was spreading the gospel of yoga. "I taught yoga classes in the evenings and weekends," he says. In 1965, with his classes overflowing, he founded the Yoga Society of Pennsylvania, which would eventually become the Kripalu Yoga Center, North America's largest yoga teacher-training center. That same year Swami A.C. Bhaktivedanta Prabhupada showed up near-penniless in New York's Tompkins Square Park and began chanting, *"Hare Krishna, Hare Rama."* Within months he'd opened America's first temple of the International Society for Krishna Consciousness, a society more popularly known as the Hare Krishnas. Nineteen sixty-five was also the year "cosmic artist" Peter Max invited his guru Swami Satchidananda to New York for a brief visit. Satchidananda liked what he saw and decided to move to the United States permanently, soon founding the Integral Yoga Institute and, in 1986, opening the Light of Truth Universal Shrine ("Yogaville") in rural Virginia. His boldface acolytes included Allen Ginsberg, Jeff Goldblum and Carole King. Actor Liev Schreiber lived at a Satchidananda ashram as a teenager.

It wasn't all one-way traffic. Westerners were heading east in droves, too, part of some grand, informal cultural-exchange program. In 1967 a professor by the name of Richard Alpert went to India on a spiritual journey, having been fired from his job at Harvard four years earlier for allegedly giving psilocybin to his undergraduates. In India he crossed paths with another American pilgrim, a strapping young streak of southern California promise named Michael Riggs. By age eighteen Riggs had become disillusioned with the monotony and materialism of suburban Western life and had headed east, throwing himself into solitary retreat. He emerged with unflinching devotion to God and a new name: Bhagavan Das. He also slapped a new name on Alpert: Ram Dass.

Elvis Presley got on board, too, in his 1967 vehicle *Easy Come, Easy Go* (not his worst picture, but about as Late Elvis as Early Elvis gets). It's the Summer of Love and the King happens to stumble across a commune of proto-hippies in the middle of a far-out yoga class. The inevitable ensues: a musical number called "Yoga Is as Yoga Does." And yoga wasn't just for the good guys. In September 1966 *Time* magazine reported on former Nazi Rudolf Hess and his life inside Spandau prison: "Hess, for the most part, lies on the floor of his 7-by-10-ft. cell, clad in grey shirt, brown corduroys and wooden clogs, and practices yoga."[2]

Although B-list movies and brownshirts sure didn't hurt, it would take another level of celebrity entirely to bring all things Eastern squarely into the mainstream. "When the Beatles went to India and became fans of Transcendental Meditation that had a huge ripple effect," says Syman, by way of understatement. While it was a whirl-wind romance, the Beatles' fling with the Maharishi Mahesh Yogi did more to establish meditation and yoga as the de rigueur flower power pastime than anything that had come before. The Beatles met the Maharishi at the London Hilton in August 1967. A few days later they were off to Bangor, Wales, to attend the Maharishi's weekend "initiation" conference. By early 1968 the Fab Four were guests at his ashram in Rishikesh, India, learning the intricate art of meditation, which the Maharishi said they had done extremely well. Mick Jagger, Marianne Faithful, Donovan, Mia Farrow and others soon followed.

The cozy atmosphere of the commune soon curdled, however, leading to one of the most notorious dust-ups of the free-love era. Ringo Starr was the first to fold, on a plane back to London with his wife, Maureen, just ten days after signing on to the mystic's tran-scendental trip. "It was just like Butlins," he supposedly told a reporter on his return, likening the atmosphere to the enforced jol-lity of the English family vacation resort chain he'd worked in as a young musician.[3] By May 1968 the rest of the Beatles had left

Rishikesh as well. "We believe in meditation, but not the Maharishi and his scene. But that's a personal mistake we made in public," John Lennon conceded a few weeks later on *The Tonight Show* with Johnny Carson.[4]

What went wrong? Conventional wisdom has it the Beatles became disillusioned when the Maharishi made sexual advances to Mia Farrow. However, the prestigious spiritualist Deepak Chopra, a former Maharishi disciple and friend of the late George Harrison, insists the Maharishi objected to the Beatles' drug use.[5] Either way, the Fab Four had fled, disillusioned and dispirited. Luckily for their fans, this tumultuous chapter was also a highly creative one. Lennon, McCartney and Harrison composed many of the songs that make up *The White Album* and *Abbey Road* at the ashram, including "Dear Prudence," written for Mia Farrow's sister, and the snarky "Sexy Sadie," about the guru himself. Originally "Maharishi," the title was changed by John Lennon to avoid potential litigation. "I was just using the situation to write a song, rather calculatingly but also to

---

The Beatles' First Break-Up

A sampling of headlines following the Beatles' split from the Maharishi Mahesh Yogi.

"Beatles Cut Ties to Maharishi"
The Washington Post, May 17, 1968

"Maharishi Yogi Turns Other Cheek to the Beatles' Slur"
Los Angeles Times, May 17, 1968

"Yogi Takes Loss of Beatles Calmly"
The Washington Post, May 24, 1968

"Beatles Moved by New Spirit"
(About the group's attempts to "contact" their late manager and close friend Brian Epstein during seances.)
The Washington Post, June 8, 1968

express what I felt. I was leaving the Maharishi with a bad taste," Lennon said during a 1980 *Playboy* interview.[6]

The reverberations from those brief, halcyon days left an indelible mark. The Beatles gave Eastern mysticism instant cachet, and the conventional culture soon followed their lead, choosing to interpret yoga largely as a drug-free high, a transcendental tonic for an increasingly toxic world. And as a tonic it came not a moment too soon. By the end of 1968 the United States had suffered through the assassinations of Robert Kennedy and Martin Luther King, through widespread protests against the Vietnam War and through violent clashes between activists and police at the Democratic National Convention in Chicago. Canadian culture was also in upheaval—with the help of some Americans. Canada did not support the war in Vietnam and thus became the American draft dodger's destination of choice. An estimated fifty thousand American war resisters immigrated across the border to Canada during the sixties and early seventies, including novelist William Gibson. Canadian protests usually came without the attendant violence of the American protests, with one notable exception: In June 1968, on the eve of a general election, supporters of Quebec independence threw bottles and rocks at new prime minister Pierre Trudeau during a Montreal parade, yelling, *"Trudeau au Poteau"* ("Trudeau to the gallows"). Trudeau impressed the electorate by refusing to take cover, likely contributing to a significant majority for his Liberal Party the next day.

Despite all the upheavals in the West, or perhaps because of them, the gurus kept coming. In 1968 B.K.S. Iyengar's *Light on Yoga* was published in the United States and became an instant classic. Many yogis still refer to it as the bible of serious asana practice. Also in 1968 the Sikh Yogi Bhajan immigrated to the United States and introduced Kundalini yoga to the masses through his Healthy, Happy, Holy Organization (3HO). And it all came to a head (or head shop, at least) in 1969, in a tiny, rain-soaked field in upstate New York, when Swami Satchidananda was chosen to give the opening speech at the seminal Woodstock music and arts festival. "My beloved brothers and sisters," Satchidananda began, echoing Vivekananda's powerful introduction to the Western world at the

Chicago Parliament of the World's Religions seventy years earlier, "I am overwhelmed with joy to see the entire youth of America gathered here in the name of music."

Satchidananda would have been lucky to see anything through the haze of pot smoke. Certainly Vivekananda would have been shocked, as many yoga purists were, to see just how seamlessly yoga had merged with the drug scene. A few years earlier the practice had seemed somehow above drugs, as if yoga could provide something that made drugs unnecessary. Offering the best example of using yoga as an antidote to the excesses of hedonism was Yogi Bhajan, whose 3HO began a drug-rehab program after Bhajan recognized how many young people were using drugs to experience higher consciousness. The program's essential message, according to Syman, was that "yoga is better than drugs." And let's not forget that the Beatles went to India in part to escape the trappings of the drug culture. Ostensibly, anyway. "I hope the fans will take up meditation instead of drugs," Ringo Starr supposedly said in 1967. Three years later John Lennon was saying about LSD: "I must have had a thousand trips. I used to just eat it all the time."[7] For others the prevalence of drugs was a way into the practice. "Yoga became much more attractive in the seventies, where people were getting into marijuana and LSD, and they were opening up to whole new areas of life that they never knew before," says Amrit Desai, former head of Kripalu Yoga Center. This emerging group, the hippies, "were really disenchanted with the society and with the culture and focus on the money and power," Desai adds.

As the sixties became the seventies, westerners continued their infatuation with yoga, gurus and getting high one way or another. By 1970 Ram Dass had returned from his quests in India and was touring college campuses with his new book, *Be Here Now*, based on his experiences with Bhagavan Das. It soon became another Age of Aquarius mystical must-read. Also in 1970, the monk and yogi Swami Rama shot to fame by demonstrating to researchers at the prestigious Menninger Foundation his ability, among other tricks, to stop his heart and to voluntarily maintain production of various brain-wave patterns, all while hooked up to a battery of instruments. In 1971 the guru Baba Hari Dass, who has maintained a vow of silence since 1952, took up residence in Santa Cruz, California, and began passing on his wisdom to westerners via scribbled messages. (His Post-it budget was easily the highest of the new gurus.) By mid-decade both Pattabhi Jois and T.K.V. Desikachar, disciples of the great master Krishnamacharya, had toured the West with their brand of yoga. Then there was Swami Muktananda, who came to the United States and launched Siddha yoga in 1970, and Joyce Green, a Jewish Brooklyn housewife who in 1973 had a vision from Jesus and reinvented herself as "Ma," an ashram leader and yoga teacher. Finally, there was Guru Maharaj Ji, the baby-faced guru whose meteoric rise began in 1971 with the founding of his Divine Light Mission.

There needed to be a record of all these comings and goings. And in May 1975, through the efforts of the California Yoga Teachers Association, *Yoga Journal* came into being. Although it's now the worldwide yoga community's undisputed voice of authority, published in China, Russia, Spain, Italy, Thailand, Hong Kong and Brazil, its inception was much less auspicious. The association printed just three hundred copies of the first ten-page edition. But the attitude was already there. "From the very beginning, *Yoga Journal* was backed by people who were very seriously interested in yoga. "Yoga missionaries, they called themselves," says *Journal* publisher John Abbott, who bought the magazine in 1998. Early articles focused almost exclusively on yoga practice and yoga figures, such as the May/June 1976 edition featuring cover-guru Satchidananda and the cover line "Swami Satchidananda, Man of Peace." "You will find traces of that magazine in the present magazine," Abbott says, noting how much the magazine has changed.[8] Then again it had to change. Yoga was changing. It was trying to survive the eighties.

When New Age Was the Rage

The sixties and seventies had been a defining, iconic time for Western yoga, a golden age. But as the eighties dawned the summers of love were a fading memory. The pot smoke, incense and patchouli of an earlier generation had wafted away. It was 1981 and the biggest song on the radio was Olivia Newton-John's "Let's Get Physical," the anthem for the new "fitness craze" that was sweeping the world.

For some, physical fitness was a "positive addiction," a remedy for the riots, disruptions and corruptions of the sixties and seventies. Having mostly failed to transform the culture, these young urban professionals now attempted to transform their bodies. They switched their yoga mats for the NordicTrack and spent big bucks on fitness equipment, gym memberships and crash diets—all to feed a rampant new obsession with health, beauty, youthfulness and sex appeal. The times belonged to step-aerobics, Jazzercise and Jane Fonda, whose juggernaut 1982 exercise video Jane Fonda's *Workout* created a second career for the already successful actress. Clad in a leotard and leg warmers, Fonda represented a new ideal of feminine beauty—jock chic, strong and healthy, and oozing sex appeal. "Today, health is beauty," top modeling agent Eileen Ford told *Time* magazine in 1982.[9] In an article detailing an era of "enlightened narcissism," Ford described the eighties look as "a firm body, healthy hair and skin, and a look of serene determination in the eyes." *The New York Times* reported on the movement's boldfaced proponents. "At 6 A.M. any weekday morning (7 A.M. on Sundays) San Vincente Boulevard from Barrington Avenue to the Pacific Ocean is full of jogging agents, actors and producers," gushed a March 1983 article. "Regulars include Elliott Gould, Valerie Harper, former California Governor Jerry Brown (who was once accompanied by his secret service escort), Arnold Schwarzenegger, and Meredith Baxter Birney."[10]

The fitness movement spawned some unlikely megastars. Richard Simmons was just another chubby kid growing up in New Orleans when he found an anonymous note addressed to him. "It said, 'Dear Richard, you're very funny, but fat people die young. Please don't die,'" recalls Simmons.[11] He didn't die. Instead he lost 130 pounds—and turned his dieting success into a career, launching a hit 1982 television exercise program called *The Richard Simmons Show.* The show and subsequent media attention made him a millionaire.

It was the eighties. Greed was good. But materialism wasn't making a comeback with everyone. Another segment of the population played out their lives far away from all the junk bonds, shoulder pads and cocaine. For them it was all about birthstones and dream weavers, crystals and channeling. These were the New Agers. While the New Age movement had been coalescing for at least two decades, it took until the early eighties for it to hit the mainstream. It remained lodged there for over a decade. Although the movement filled the culture's ever-present need to "connect" with something larger, it didn't spring from a holy text or dogma, nor was it passed down by a formal clergy. Their beliefs were a smorgasbord. New Agers often grafted new ideas onto their pre-existing religious or spiritual affiliations, taking only what worked and discarding the rest. In was a shaggy kind of pseudo-spirituality, an attempt to Get with God on your own terms. In other words, it had a lot in common with yoga.

Perhaps because of these similarities, the early New Age movement threatened to render much of yoga irrelevant. Copies of *Yoga Journal* are a time capsule of this anxious period. As early as 1980 the magazine was pondering the shift. "Today, the question of a new age ... is more important than ever," one article read. "For without some major changes in the next decade, we may not have the luxury of speculating about the 1990's."[12] According to publisher John Abbott, the eighties version of *Yoga Journal* was "very much a New Age yoga magazine, meaning that about a third of the content was dedicated to yoga and two-thirds to other New Age lifestyle issues. We'd write about crystals." That ended when he took over the magazine in 1998. "My wish from the beginning was that *Yoga Journal* be a yoga magazine," he says. "We didn't need to do 'Conquering Your Fears through Trapeze Flying.'"

Yoga didn't seem to stand a chance. It had been sidelined by the overlapping ideals of the New Age movement and shunted aside by Reagan, Rambo and a string of muscular, masculine Me Generation heroes. To many, yoga had become passé. But the practice was too resilient to just disappear. As had happened endless times before, yoga needed to be reborn. No longer viable as a counterculture escape, yoga slowly re-emerged as a stress-relief regimen, a de rigueur appendage to both the fitness and New Age movements. Thus began the second (and shortest) phase of "modern yoga."

In the late eighties busy boomers began looking for ways to counteract all that heavy lifting of a few years earlier. Studies had revealed that moderate exercise produced as many health benefits as more strenuous workouts, while some high-impact exercise was found to be counterproductive, even dangerous. Jim Fixx wrote *The Complete Book of Running*, the movement's must-have read. In 1984, aged just fifty-two, Fixx died of a massive heart attack—right after his daily run. Marathon runners were also dropping dead of heart attacks. Many people abandoned the sport altogether. When researchers discovered some high-impact aerobics caused stress fractures and other injuries, even Jane Fonda began concentrating her energies elsewhere.

The early eighties had also been a time of insatiable and conspicuous consumption, and by the late eighties a collective mid-life crisis seemed to be seeping in. Even some Masters of the Universe, as Tom Wolfe famously described the eighties' financial and social elite, were wringing their hands over the orgies of materialism and greed they'd been privy to. Yoga presented a way to neutralize, or at least to *appear* to neutralize, those pangs and proclivities. It offered a connection to something greater and more meaningful. It was the newest form of detox, "a way to get fitness and also get stress-relief and to discover some of these other, possibly spiritual dimensions," says Trisha Lamb, formerly of the Yoga Research and Education Center.

By the mid-eighties the New Agers who weren't already into yoga were discovering just how much the two movements had in common, and how easily yogic concepts such as meditation and natural healing could be reinterpreted to fit a New Age worldview. Shirley MacLaine was the most high profile of these metaphysical Fellow-Travelers. The actress had been a dedicated yogini and follower of Kolkata-based guru Bikram Choudhury since the early sixties, even encouraging Choudhury to bring his practice stateside, which he did in 1973. Then MacLaine had a spiritual awakening that kicked off a years-long search for self-discovery, which she described in her 1983 bestselling book, *Out on a Limb*. MacLaine's search, which established her as the eighties go-to New Age celebrity, opened her up to the prototypical New Age beliefs: UFO encounters, trance mediums, reincarnation, astral projection and the like. She kept up her yoga practice, all the while shrugging off any suggestion that she was the leader of a new movement. "I'm not a high priestess of New Age concepts. I'm just a human being trying to find some answers about what we're doing here," she told *Time* magazine in 1987.[13]

The injection of New Age ideals into yoga and the antics that followed often hurt yoga's credibility. *Time* ran an article in August 1987 titled "A New Age Dawning," about disparate groups across the United States gathering one Sunday morning at the behest of José Argüelles, an art historian and follower of Mayan culture. Argüelles' examination of ancient Mayan calendars led him to believe that the "materialistic" world would end on that day, when three planets lined up with the new moon "unless 144,000 true believers gathered in various 'sacred sites' around the world and 'resonated' sufficiently to bring on a new age of peace and harmony," according to the article. "As the darkness dissolved, yoga practitioners began a series of alarming birdlike maneuvers."[14]

The problem was that yoga wasn't attracting new blood. The people practicing yoga were by and large from the same pool they'd come from for years; postwar baby boomers who had embraced yoga from the beginning, rediscovered it or never left it. If yoga were to survive it would need a kick-start, a youthful, sexy, marketable edge. It seemed unlikely.

Dr. Dean Ornish probably had little inkling of how much he was changing the course of Western yoga when he published his bestselling book *Dr. Dean Ornish's Program for Reversing Heart Disease* in 1990. A long-time disciple of Swami Satchidananda, Ornish had a hunch that the rigorous yoga and strict vegetarianism at the heart of his guru's practice might help with heart disease, one of the Western world's biggest killers. His hunch was right. His now-famous studies showed that yoga, combined with diet, meditation and group support, can reverse heart disease.[15] The notion that something as benign as yoga could have restorative powers was not easy for the medical establishment to accept. "When I first began conducting research twenty-three years ago, we had to refer to yoga as 'stress management techniques,'" Ornish told *Yoga Journal*. "'We can't refer to a study that includes yoga—what are we going to tell patients, that we're referring them to a swami?' Since then, yoga has achieved much greater acceptance within American medicine."[16]

That's an understatement. The media were soon full of stories about Western medicine's embrace of yoga, meditation and stress-relief practices. In November 1996 *The New York Times* reported on the number of American HMOs offering alternative medicine as part of their health insurance plans, detailing an announcement by Oxford Health Plans that it would become the first large medical insurer to have a network of alternative-care providers such as yoga instructors, acupuncturists and naturopaths. Of course, this was also good business, a response to consumer demand, the article noted. "Managed-care organizations are competing bitterly with each other and are looking for every kind of marketing tool they can find to get people to sign up with them," said George D. Lundberg, editor of the *Journal of the American Medical Association*.[17] Another *Times* article from August 1996 asserted that "Relaxation Method May Aid Health," citing a study that showed patients assigned to practice Transcendental Meditation had blood pressure reductions similar to those commonly achieved with antihypertensive drugs.[18] And another factor was at play, says Trisha Lamb. "One of the primary ways that yoga has made its way into the medical community is through physicians, nurses, wives of physicians and husbands of physicians saying, 'Oh, there's great potential, great *untapped* potential here.'"

This trend soon linked up with another burgeoning yoga craze, the athleticization of yoga, what Lamb calls the "'no pain, no gain,' if-you-don't-sweat-it's-not-good-for-you" type of yoga. It came to be popularly known as Power yoga, from the title of Beryl Bender Birch's breakthrough 1995 book that brought the sweaty, stringent Ashtanga yoga style to prominence. In February 1995 *Yoga Journal* ran a cover article titled "Power Yoga" about Ashtanga, describing it as "yoga aerobics with a meditative flair" and the "hip new way to burn off calories, sculpt your buns, and sweat away the flab around your waist."[19]

The natural habitat of these sweat- and strain-obsessed yogis were the gyms and health clubs that now dotted the Western landscape. Newspaper stories began appearing about this new, brawny yoga rolling up its mat, blowing out the candles and moving into a gym *right around the corner from you!* All of this appealed to an aging population, says Lamb, "[that] large cohort of baby-boomers who are reaching middle-age and not able to jog without damaging their knees." Soon the corporations started taking notice. "In the early nineties the hot topic was yoga in the workplace," Lamb says. "Now, it's just standard to have yoga in the workplace. All the major corporations offer yoga classes or offer discounted access to them."

By the mid-nineties an unprecedented yogic groundswell was underway. Yoga had sprung from the ghettos of the niche magazines onto the style and fashion pages of seemingly every paper in America. The third—and rowdiest—stage of modern yoga had begun. In many ways it was a commingling of all the manifestations of yoga that had come before. Rather than shed its skin entirely each time, yoga retained what worked and kept on moving. It was athletic yet low impact. It could rejuvenate and restore. It was mentally and spiritually nourishing. What better way to stave off that heart attack *and* get a great butt! Old faces jumped aboard the new yoga train. In 1993 Jane Fonda, the celebrated Queen of Fitness Videos, who had abandoned the "burn" a few years earlier, came out with a new product—*Jane Fonda's Yoga Exercise Workout.* A year later Ali MacGraw dropped *Ali MacGraw: Yoga Mind & Body.*

But to truly crown yoga's new wave of popularity, to anoint it fully acceptable to the mainstream, there would need to be new mascots. And what this new crop of high priests and priestesses did to yoga's profile makes the Beatles looks like rank amateurs.

Soul Train

A March 1998 article in *The New York Times* (which by this stage was starting to look like a satellite office of *Yoga Journal*) asked us to "imagine Madonna in the most unlikely position she could take." Sitting at home, in front of the TV? Hardly. The Pop Princess was instead "lying face up on the floor in a yoga pose known as the corpse, crying uncontrollably," the article continued. " 'As my body was opening up and I was going into places that had been locked for so many years, it was releasing emotional things,' " the Immaculate One shared. " 'I'd do a forward bend and tears would come to my eyes. I'd sort of get embarrassed and think, "why is this happening to me?" But I realized that I was going through a catharsis.'" Madonna explained that although she'd tried yoga just to stay in shape after the birth of her daughter, Lourdes, she had now found "deeper lessons."[20]

The risqué posturing and bawdy button pushing was out. The Material Girl was now the Spiritual Girl. And the best part? It was all because of another celebrity! According to *Women's Fitness and Health* magazine, it was Sting who introduced Madonna to yoga through his guru, the handily named Danny Paradise. "One day when I was working with Sting she came over to his apartment and watched some of the practice. Trudie Styler (Sting's wife) told me later that from that moment on she [Madonna] wanted to learn Yoga," Paradise was quoted as saying.[21]

Whether the Mother of Reinvention's latest incarnation as über-yogini was standard celebrity navel-gazing narcissism or real spiritual catharsis didn't seem to matter. Nobody cared *how* the King of Pain found yoga. The point is they had, and many more people would because of them. Younger people, too, as the muscular, precise Ashtanga method Madonna and Sting favored appealed to this much-coveted demographic. Barnaby Harris owns the Fuck Yoga store in New York. (Don't worry, we'll come back to this.) "All my mom's friends were doing yoga in the sixties and seventies," Harris recalls. "Nobody said anything. And then what happened was Madonna.... I guarantee you that if Sting, Madonna, and Willem Dafoe were Jazzercising, then none of this would have occurred."[22]

It's true that the yoga world was beginning to resemble a giant *Us* magazine photo spread, as stars nudged their yoga mats aside to make room for one another in class and clustered together at yoga studio openings and parties. It was perfect fodder for our celebrity- and body-obsessed culture, fueling the enduring myth of a tight-knit entertainment "community," a utopia of creative cohorts and costars all wanting nothing but the best for one another, and now doing it through yoga.

There was a nexus for all this remarkable munificence: the Jivamukti Yoga Center in downtown New York. The Jivamukti method (*jivamukti* is a Sanskrit word meaning "liberation while living") was created in 1984 by business and life partners Sharon Gannon and David Life. Having plied their trade as performers in New York's East Village, the pair decided they could be of "better service," as Gannon puts it, teaching yoga. The beginnings were humble for the Jivamukti Yoga Society, as it was called then. "We started in our apartment. It was just people coming over," Gannon recalls, until "the apartment got too full of people." The first Jivamukti Yoga Center was opened in 1989, on Second Avenue in the city's East Village, with Diane Keaton as the first Big Name. Word of the hot new yoga center soon got around, and business boomed. By 1998 Gannon and Life had relocated Jivamukti to a larger space on Lafayette Street, still in the East Village. Soon celebrity, spirituality and prosperity were colliding regularly and fabulously, quickly etching Jivamukti into the public consciousness as the Yoga Studio to the Stars. "It wasn't our intention to have some large, successful yoga center, even a worldwide movement of any sort," says Life. "All we did was try to share what we knew with people who were interested. What happened to it, I think, is more a product of the potency of that message than it is of planning."[23]

Jivamukti parties made the Oscars look like a check-cutting ceremony at the local recreational center. In March 1998 *Entertainment Weekly* reported on a "klieg-lit soiree" at Jivamukti that attracted Sting, along with Willem Dafoe and Mike D of the Beastie Boys.[24] Meanwhile, sweating it out in Jivamukti classes were the usual yogaratti; funnyman Steve Martin, hip-hop mogul Russell Simmons, thespians Mary Stuart Masterson and Sarah Jessica Parker and supermodel Christy Turlington. "Celebrities come to these practices for the same reasons anybody would; they're looking for happiness, they don't have any ulterior motives," says Life. And while he rejects the Studio-to-the-Stars label, he concedes that celebrities have been an important part of Jivamukti's success: "It may be not such a great calling card here, but we've found it very useful in making inroads and opening doors in countries where there's no knowledge of these practices." Gannon says that the "rock stars" who come to Jivamukti "are the most disciplined hard-working people that I know. To be associated with a disciplined, hard-working person whose aim is to uplift the world, I think it's a compliment."

It seems Madonna may have gotten a little too disciplined about her yoga, admitting at one point that her yoga practice bordered on unhealthy obsession. "I could've been a member of Cirque du Soleil. It got to the point where I didn't have a glass of wine and I had to go to bed early because everything was around my yoga," *People* magazine's website reported her as saying.[25] And the monster she helped create rolled on. The speed and rapacity of yoga's growth startled seasoned vets such as James Barkan, owner and director of the Barkan Method yoga school, who began practicing in the late seventies, when yoga was still on the fringes. "I never foresaw this many people getting into yoga ten years ago, fifteen years ago," Barkan says. "In the year 2000 it really started to hit mainstream America."

The new millennium had blown up a perfect yogic storm. Westerners were reveling in unprecedented wealth, fueled by the new dot-com sector. More people now had more time and more money to throw at yoga, which had become available in more and more places. And the rise of "yoga chic" meant that this time it wasn't just the baby boomers and aging hippies who were facing east. "Yoga went public," says futurist Barry Minkin. "TV, movie stars, shows about yoga ..."[26]

Yoga had become a bona fide social phenomenon, a global cultural juggernaut that cut across lines of age, gender, race, class and sexual orientation, enveloping everyone from mothers to money managers. A 2008 study commissioned by *Yoga Journal* found that 15.8 million Americans—6.9 percent of the adult American population—regularly practiced some version of yoga.[27] A 2005 study reveals 5.5 percent of Canadian adults or 1.4 million people practicing yoga, an increase of 15 percent from the previous year and of almost 50 percent from 2003.[28] In 2005 more Australians practiced yoga than played Aussie rules football, the cherished national pastime.[29] Yoga has integrated itself into almost every aspect of modern culture, according to Trisha Lamb. "It's not just down at the local corner yoga studio like it was twenty years ago; it's in health clubs, it's in gyms. It's in the workplace, in prisons, even in judges' chambers. It's in nursing homes. It's in the public and private schools. It's in the universities. It's in almost every aspect of our culture today, and in positive ways," she says. "It's having a positive transformative effect everywhere it's practiced."

In May 2006 Jivamukti was once again moving to bigger digs. The plush new space in New York's Union Square has become the cornerstone of what Jivamukti's publicist calls the studio's yoga lifestyle. As well as yoga classes there's a vegan café where "reality sandwiches" and "salvation salads" are served. And of course there are fabulous parties. At the requisite glittering opening soiree, the usual cast of celebrities greeted David Life and Sharon Gannon with bows. "Look at me, I'm seventy-five and I look great!" said Sting.[30] (He's actually fifty-four.) Russell Simmons and his now ex-wife Kimora Lee danced to the music. Elizabeth Berkley (*Showgirls!*) was radiant in her bright pink wrap. Uma Thurman sat with her brother Declan, tapping away at her cell phone.

That's how it all looked to the reporter from the *New York Observer,* anyway. I didn't witness any of this personally. I was standing out on the street. Although I'd been making a documentary about the yoga business for the past two years and already had been granted access to many of the people inside, I hadn't been "accredited" for this event. So I stood outside, with a swarm of paparazzi and autograph hunters, trying to buttonhole celebrities as they walked by. I was brushed aside by Sting. Uma was too busy airkissing Matthew Modine to stop for me. Baron Baptiste and I might have had a word, but just as I approached, he slid past security, eager to sidestep a brewing skirmish. A dashiki-clad desperado was badgering a harried-looking publicity flak, hectoring her to "check the list again." I caught the eye of a security guard hired specifically to keep the likes of the desperado away. The guard was of the old school— weary, working class. His look said it all: "You *gotta* be kidding me."

Rise of the Yoga Mogul

There's no doubt that for some, yoga is a calling, an opportunity to serve others in service of oneself. For others the call is more like the bell that opens the New York Stock Exchange. There's moola to be made in yoga. Lots of it. The century-long marriage between this storied Eastern discipline and the great Western religion of commercialism has entered its most blissful phase. High-priced Canadian yoga outfitter lululemon (the lower case "l" is deliberate) made sales of $148.9 million in 2006.[31] The company went public in July 2007, and in three months lululemon's stock had climbed from $25 to $60. In 1999 supermodel Christy Turlington joined forces with Puma to create clothing and accessories aimed at what she described as "mind/body sports" like yoga. Her cotton tank top will set you back $80. The "Christy" Yoga Mat Bag, designed by Turlington's friend Marc Jacobs, costs around $350. Thankfully, some proceeds go to charity.

Yoga is an ad agency's dream platform, regarded as both inspirational and accessible, a perfect vehicle to sell everything from laptops to Land Cruisers. That's a big shift from previous generations, according to author Stefanie Syman. "Before, people were able to sell yoga successfully but weren't interested or weren't able to use yoga to sell other things," she says. "Now yoga is available to market other things that have nothing to do with it." Major brands such as Adidas and Nike have discovered whole new markets: yoga mats, yoga pants, yoga hoodies, yoga unitards, yoga headbands, yoga straps, yoga visors, yoga blocks, yoga bras, yoga duffel bags, even yoga shoes, despite that almost all yoga is practiced barefoot.

In the United States some yogis don't balk at paying upward of $27 for a single class, while the average cost usually falls somewhere between $15 and $20. Even at the low-end a regular yoga practice can be a costly pursuit. "To pay $17 for a yoga class, that really bothers me," says journalist and yogini Elizabeth Kadetsky. "It is very troubling that it's a very narrow cross-section of society that you see at yoga classes." That narrow cross-section was laid out in *Yoga Journal*'s 2008 study, which found that three-quarters of yogis were women, seven out of ten had a postsecondary education and almost half came from households with an income over $75,000, well above the norm. In other words, yoga is elitist.

Present-day yogis are praying at an altar of entrepreneurship and sheer chutzpah that has seen $850 Gucci yoga mats fly off the shelves. "When you think about perhaps 18 million people in the United States doing yoga, if you just throw out a theoretical $1000 a year for classes, books and mats and clothes, etc., that becomes an

$18 billion business," futurist and economic consultant Barry Minkin says. "That's more sales than Coca-Cola does in the United States or McDonald's does in the United States or Gillette does in the United States." In the United Kingdom it's a similar story. In 2003 yogis spent an estimated £670 million ($1.3 billion) on yoga and other "spiritual spending."[32]

The physical practice itself has become comically commodified. Witness the countless yoga hybrids ("supermarket yoga") that have sprung up, each designed to fill unimaginably tiny niches and sate yet-discovered whims. There's Doggie yoga (Doga), Smoking yoga (Smoga), Christian yoga, Rowga (yoga for rowers), Yoga Afloat® ("a comprehensive aquatic yoga program"), Canoe yoga (an uniquely Canadian blend of canoeing and yoga), Golf yoga (hence the "Body Golf Basic Yoga for Golfers" DVD) and even a yoga-centric comic strip, *Gangsta Yoga with DJ Dog*. "With the short attention spans, people need a new yoga every other month. And there's somebody out there that's ready to give it to them," says Minkin. "The purists must be really, really upset with some of this that's going on. Particularly that a number of them are successful!"

Indeed, purists have long feared that yoga's phenomenal growth has planted the seeds of its own destruction. Constantly diluting yoga's original purpose through endless commercialism and reinvention may strip yoga of any meaning at all, they say. The goal of yoga, after all, is detachment and enlightenment. Much in today's yoga scene seems designed only to enlighten us of our wallets and detach us from our savings. "When any practice gets institutionalized, there's definitely a dumbing down in some circles. There's a gross, slick aspect," says Rodney Yee. He fears yoga may soon become "so much a business that it loses its real interest as an inward practice."[33] Of course, this should be taken with a grain of salt. Yee has over thirty yoga DVDs on the market, boasts the compulsory celebrity clientele, including Demi Moore and designer Donna Karan, and spends much of his time on the lucrative yoga conference circuit.

Conferences have become a lucrative adjunct to the mainstream yoga industry. *Yoga Journal* got into the business in 1994, holding a single event that year. During the 2007–2008 season, *Yoga Journal* held five such events, each offering an eclectic mix of elasticity and enlightenment. A four-day pass usually sets you back over $900. The conferences attract the rock stars of yoga: Rodney Yee, Baron Baptiste, Sharon Gannon, Shiva Rea, Cyndi Lee. The atmosphere borders on evangelical. Return attendees (many of them yoga teachers themselves) jostle for a few rapturous minutes at the feet of their chosen gurus. Their interactions are uncynical. "He's so humble, and people constantly shower him with praise," one attendee said to a *New York Times* reporter of Baron Baptiste. "I like his public persona," another gushed about Rodney Yee. "He's not threatening, like some yoga teachers."[34]

Then there are yoga "retreats." These are a little more open to interpretation. Usually held on some far-flung and sun-drenched shore, the retreats often present yoga combined with some other activity—rock climbing, surfing, perhaps even some good old conventional lying around. At the Dunton Hot Springs resort in Colorado, the day starts with a vigorous Ashtanga practice, followed by an organic breakfast and either a long hike through the Rocky Mountains or a soak in a natural hot spring. A week of this costs $1250. Advertisements for the "Santorini with Rusty Wells" retreat in Santorini, Greece, promise a healthy dose of Vinyasa Flow administered by yoga "legend" Rusty Wells, along with a "big taste of Greek culture." That week will cost you $1399, transport, alas, not included. "The Spiritual Wisdom of the Andes" yoga retreat in Cuzco, Peru, is another big seller. The program features outdoor solar medicinal baths, a crystal bed for "healing" and visits to "sacred sites," including those of Cuzco and Machu Picchu.[35]

Closer to home, I decide to visit the annual Omega Yoga Conference in New York City, operated by the Omega Institute for Holistic Studies in upstate New York, perhaps the most prominent New Age institution in the United States. Omega was founded in 1977 by Elizabeth Lesser and her then-husband, Dr. Stephan Rechtschaffen, typical sixties seekers who decided to form their own institute dedicated to awakening "the best in the human spirit" and providing "hope and healing for individuals and society," according to their website.[36]

I didn't exactly see the best of the human spirit on display, but perhaps I'd just come in a bum year. (Al Gore was guest speaker at the 2007 conference.) What I *did* see was commerce in full swing: joss sticks aplenty, mounds of crystal-based jewelry, countless creams and pastes, untold amounts of oils, ointments and emollients, as well as a man selling gold statues of Shiva atop a sign declaring, "We Ship Worldwide." The Omega Bookstore and Media Works showroom was a particularly fecund retail experience, packed with more self-help books and DVDs than one person could possibly devour in this or several subsequent lifetimes. Titles included *Yoga for Women, Chicken Soup for the Sister's Soul, Where Dogs Dream* and *Creative Menopause.*

I catch up with John Friend, creator of the Anusara yoga style and a guest teacher at the conference. "Everybody wants to be free. Free from pain, their suffering, their fears," he says. "I really hope everybody is here for that ultimate freedom. At the same time, there are superficial motives that we all are motivated by.... There's an entertainment factor. One guy today, the tech, said, 'Have a good show.' He wished me a good show. People come, and they don't even know me, but they want to have their photo taken with me or have my signature on something. I'm saying, 'Well, this isn't a show.' "[37]

"This is what happens in America," says Trisha Lamb. "We have this big Madison Avenue machine and if something becomes a hot topic in which a lot of Americans are interested, it's going to be exploited for merchandising."

Wandering back through the showrooms I found myself staring at a basket full of marked-down yoga goodies—an assortment of garishly colored, impishly small undergarments. I was immediately reminded of something Lamb had said to me a few months earlier. Although she worked hard to keep an even head about even the most egregious yoga trends, one product really pushed her buttons. "The one that kind of crosses the line for me is 'chakra panties,' " Lamb had told me. "What next? Where will they take it next?"

I turned over the chakra panties in my hand and decided I didn't need them after all. Besides, they wouldn't fit any human being I know.

Should it surprise us that yoga has become so commercialized? Yoga has always been a mirror of the culture—and look at the culture. Look at the houses we build. Even though the typical Western family has gotten smaller, the average new American home exceeds three thousand square feet, twice the size of an average home of 1950. Look at the cars we drive. There are more than 24 million SUVs on American roads, one for every eight licensed drivers. Witness the consumerist orgy we call Christmas. The "holiday gift giving" blitzkrieg now "officially" starts the day after Halloween, on November 1. (In the United States, Lexus has perfected a strategy that combines these two hungers. Its "December to Remember" ad campaign urged viewers to give a Lexus to a loved one, or even one-self, as a holiday gift. According to *Adweek,* the strategy worked, with Toyota claiming 10 percent of the Lexus vehicles sold that December were given as gifts.)[38]

Yes, we live in a standardized, corporatized culture where super-size does matter. Call it McWorld. And McWorld has exactly the yoga it deserves.

4

McYoga

Yoga is universal.... But don't approach yoga with a
business mind looking for worldly gain.
—SRI K. PATTABHI JOIS, QUOTED IN *YOGA + JOYFUL
LIVING* MAGAZINE

Ten years ago if you'd done an Internet search for the words *yoga franchise* (*were* we Googling ten years ago?) you wouldn't have gotten much. Try searching that phrase today and you'll get back dozens of "opportunities," from Bikram Yoga to Nava Yoga, CorePower Yoga to Progressive Power Yoga, Sunstone Yoga to Sonic Yoga. The yoga franchise, a Starbucks-style formula for financial success and karmic well-being, is just the latest example of how yoga has molded itself to meet the demands of our standardized culture. The website for Sonic Yoga's franchise ("Pure ecstasy!") encourages you to imagine yourself teaching a yoga class, "smiling in every cell of your being as you glisten with pride, compassion and energy. This is not just living, this is being alive."[1]

The undisputed kings of this new business model are Rob Wrubel and George Lichter, cofounders of Yoga Works, arguably the world's most successful yoga franchise. The boyish, sandy-haired, six-foot Wrubel and the bookish, salt-and-pepper-haired Lichter first met in 1994, at an educational software company called Knowledge

Adventure. Wrubel went on to become the first chief executive of Ask Jeeves International, a unit of the web search engine Ask Jeeves Inc. His role, according to Lichter, "was to take something hard and make it simple, put a human face on it—the face of a butler. And then make it better so everyone could use it." Wrubel then brought Lichter aboard to help keep moving the company forward. Jeeves was a huge success, with stocks soaring to more than $200 a share.

But the work was taking its toll. "We'd been on the road a lot, me international and Rob domestic, flying around, neglecting our bodies," Lichter said. By 2002 both Wrubel and Lichter had left the company, battered by the long hours, the dot-com bust and the decline of Jeeves stock. But it was in their bodies that the toll really showed. Wrubel had gained almost thirty pounds during his three years at Ask Jeeves and his blood pressure had soared. For Lichter severe headaches and persistent back and leg pain became so great that he began wearing a back brace. Yoga would open new doors in more ways than one. Both men had discovered yoga as a way to rehabilitate their bodies. A copy of Richard Hittleman's book *Yoga for Health* turned Lichter on, while Wrubel's wife encouraged him to try yoga, after he'd exhausted countless physical therapists and chiropractors. Through yoga Wrubel had gotten his weight comfortably back under 200 pounds, while his partner's back pain had become a thing of the past.

I sit down with Wrubel and Lichter inside one of the New York City Yoga Works studios. In person the pair share an easy camaraderie, a back-and-forth no doubt perfected by endless pitch-practice sessions. "The interesting part," Lichter says, glancing across at Wrubel, "is that we *weren't* sharing this." It was during one of their weekly brainstorming sessions in late 2001 that yoga came to the forefront. They were searching for a new venture, "something that might make an important contribution to society," as Wrubel puts it. "We were talking about all these ideas, from online educational services to water purifying technology for the Third World. And at one point we were looking at each other ..." Wrubel seems unsure quite how to phrase the rest of it, then continues. "And we did that funny moment where we said, 'Boy, you're looking good.'" They started comparing notes, and an idea soon took shape. "We said, 'Let's create a business where we can make great yoga accessible to many more people.' "[2]

Their initial aim was a group of studios across the United States, with perhaps eight to ten studios in each major city. They also harbored more ambitious goals, of making yoga "a permanent feature of the health-care landscape," Wrubel says. "I would love to see in every hospital, you go down the aisle and every recovering cancer patient is doing yoga in the morning. And the kids who are suffering in the critical care or the recovery areas are doing yoga." Lichter nods in agreement. "If we can get health care and medical insurance and third-party payer systems to start contributing, then that goes toward the goal of making yoga more available and affordable to everyone. That's a key trend that we think assists in democratizing yoga," he says.

But to make these lofty dreams a reality the pair needed studios. In 2003, with the early financing in place, Wrubel and Lichter bought up five struggling yoga studios across California. By 2008 Yoga Works had eighteen studios, eight in Los Angeles and five each in Orange County, California, and in New York City. Although the studios share a basic common look, George Lichter says he wants each studio to *feel* different, to reflect the community and neighborhood around them. "I think it would be a great failing in the end if our goal would create something that was devoid of that personality," he says.

The media felt differently, quickly labeling Yoga Works "McYoga" and "the Starbucks of yoga"—although it was never entirely clear if this was as an insult or a compliment. Traditional yogis, meanwhile, were openly antagonistic toward the idea of a yoga chain. "We bristle at the word *chain*. And from the first time we wrote the business description we edited that word out every time we saw it," says Rob Wrubel. "People would say, 'You're a chain,' and we'd say, 'No, we're a family of yoga schools.' "

The problem is not everyone is happy about joining the family.

The Chain Gang

The Center for Yoga was the brainchild of the American guru Ganga White, described as a yoga pioneer by *Yoga Journal* and one of the "architects of American yoga." White was just another eleven-year-old kid growing up in rural Los Angeles when he saw the word *yogi* written on a school sidewalk with chalk. Another kid told him yogis were "these guys in the Himalayas who could wave their hands and make a flower appear," White recalls. He was intrigued, and a career in yoga was born.[3]

In September 1967, having just returned from an intensive yoga retreat in India, White opened up his own yoga studio, the Center for Yoga, on Sunset Boulevard in Los Angeles. Classes were small and payment was by donation only. But the center grew quickly and by 1968 had moved to larger digs to accommodate new students. (It was in the new location in 1968 that White led what was probably the first yoga-teacher-training course in North America.) The center brought disparate yoga styles together under one roof, blending them into a new concoction called "Flow." As White gave demonstrations at be-ins and love-ins across California, big-name yogis such as Peter Sellers and Ravi Shankar took classes at his studio.

The Center for Yoga became the prototypical southern California sixties yoga studio experience, a drop-in center for go-to gurus, celebrities and philosophers. It operated independently and successfully for almost four decades, opening ashrams, pumping out teachers and maintaining an aura of integrity and tolerance. But by 2004 the Center for Yoga had become a victim of its own success: White's graduates were opening their own yoga centers, while Flow was being taught in gyms and health clubs across North America. Things spiraled downward quickly. Deeply in debt, the center, this "wonderful collection of students and instructors," as George Lichter describes them, had not only ceased to be special, it had become almost irrelevant. That's when Yoga Works swooped.

In April 2004 this storied hub of yoga shut its doors. When it reopened soon after, it was a branch of the Yoga Works "family," the Yoga Works Center for Yoga. To hear Rob Wrubel tell it, Yoga Works had done the center a favor. "It was about to go out of business. It was about to shut its doors, so the community would have lost the center completely," he says. An *LA Weekly* article about the takeover offers a different perspective. Calling the center's demise a "surrender to the corporatization of the trend it helped to create," the article detailed an unhappy scene where "teachers made warning announcements in classes, staffers quit, notes sprouted on bathroom walls, and rumors flew."[4]

"In the beginning we probably weren't well understood, and the guards were up," Lichter says. He could appreciate the cynicism, calling it "well placed." "We live in a world where we are taken apart, where we no longer feel connected to the generation before us or the generation after us, to our colleagues; we're made to fight in corporate environments, to compete; we go home sometimes and we don't know the neighbor down the hall, down the block; there is no sense of connection; everything's just processed through and then spit back out to us. We have to fight that very strongly," he says. Wrubel nods in agreement, adding that it's similar to "the way Starbucks or Wal-Mart has come in and changed the landscape of America. For some people it's good and for some people it has taken away the special features of our landscape." But the takeover happened. And according to Lichter, the bad vibes are a thing of the past. "Now it is almost like a celebration. Students that I would engage in very testy conversations with on the street corners, we're now doing yoga next to each other."

The raw numbers, meanwhile, seem to support Wrubel's assessment that Yoga Works has reinvigorated failing studios. The number of students at an Orange County studio Yoga Works took over jumped by over 50 percent in just two years. Another location in Beverly Hills had the same increase in a single year.[5] And for the purveyors of yoga accessories, the success of Yoga Works is welcome news, says Trisha Lamb. "We [the Yoga Research and Education Center] get calls from someone who wants to introduce a new project—say, aromatherapy—into the yoga studio. Well, it's very difficult for them, because there's no chain of yoga studios, so there's no central distribution point. So they'll be pleased by this," she says. Indeed, the Yoga Works lobby is stuffed with yoga paraphernalia, from T-shirts to herbal body bars, from brand-name prayer rings to

"Skidless by Yogitoes" yoga mats. But is this really what the students want?

"I have received many calls from students and teachers connected to the center, and most of them have been negative about the changes," Ganga White claimed in the *LA Weekly* article. "Yoga is in a time of great growth, change and mutation. Mutations can be evolutionary or detrimental. I hope [the Center for Yoga] maintains the broad and open-minded perspective for which it has become known and respected." George Lichter remains philosophical: "The yoga community is realizing that everything is changing, and I think what we're doing is part of that change. But given our commitment to yoga this looks like a pretty good result."

Costly Exercise

Sunstone Yoga is a chain of studios offering a wide menu of hot and power yoga classes. In 2006 Sunstone became one of the first independent yoga studios to try its hand at franchising. By April 2008 Sunstone had sold twenty franchise opportunities.

Sunstone assures potential franchisees that the "efficiencies" of its business model deliver a "world-class fitness experience at a small business price." But if you're wondering how much that price might be, there's no immediate answer. To receive further "valuable information" you're asked to submit a contact form via email.

Given how difficult and complicated it can be to keep a room heated to hot yoga levels, it *could* be quite pricey. To properly outfit a studio with a suitable hot yoga heating and ventilation system might cost as much as $94,000, according to one website. Running that system won't be free, either. Some estimates go as high as $17,000 a month.[6] A love of yoga will get you a long way toward owning your own studio, but deep pockets will get you farther.

I decide to attend the opening of the first Yoga Works studio in New York, located on the second floor of a nondescript building on the

Upper West Side. The space is clean and welcoming, the studios airy and open, the employees scrubbed and friendly. And unflappable. I'm standing in the lobby listening to them bat away the barrage of interested callers ("Hello, Yoga Works! Can you hold?!") when one employee puts the phone down with a guffaw. An angry caller has just hung up on her. "He said we're turning yoga into a commercial circus!" she says. The other employees chuckle.

Much of this fast-gathering yogic throng is here to take a free class with renowned yogi Alan Finger. Finger, like Baron Baptiste, is a member of yoga's few Western royal families. His father Kavi Yogiraj Mani Finger, South Africa's most eminent yogi, created an ashram in his Johannesburg home, where he also taught his teenage son yoga. By the early sixties, young Alan was teaching, too. Together father and son went on to create their own yoga style known as ISHTA (Integrated System of Hatha, Tantra and Ayurveda). Alan Finger came to the United States in 1975, founding Yoga Works in Los Angeles. In 1993 Finger moved east to New York and started Yoga Zone, one of the first recognizable yoga brands, and an empire that Finger lorded over for more than a decade. He was lead instructor on the *Yoga Zone* instructional DVD series, host of the *Yoga Zone* television show and coauthor of the books *Yoga Zone: An Introduction to Yoga* and *Yoga Zone: Yoga for Life*. In 1999 Yoga Zone became Be Yoga.

The *Los Angeles Times* called Finger "the first yoga millionaire," and he's often described as one of the industry's savviest businessmen.[7] (Faint praise perhaps, considering how notoriously little business savvy some studio owners exhibit.) "Everyone always assumes that I am the financial and yogi business guy that made it. I've never done any of it! I've always had partners," Finger tells me, as we sit down cross-legged in one of his studios.[8] Finger's latest partnership has brought his yoga journey full circle. In summer 2004 George Lichter and Rob Wrubel acquired Be Yoga. What started at Yoga Works across the United States three decades before was once again Yoga Works—although in a much different form.

Finger is a calming presence, one of the few yogis I've met who really seems to radiate the calm and openness he espouses. Unlike Ganga White, Finger says selling out to Wrubel and Lichter has been a relief. "To have these guys come in and bring all of their expertise, and the financial end of it into it, really allows us, as yogis, to teach well and do what my vision was all along. So I'm really happy about it," he says. When I tell him what the irate caller said to the receptionist earlier he merely chuckles. "It's not a commercial circus. In fact, it's adding stability to the yoga, because it's very hard to have stability if there is no financial stability. So to me, for example, I can really go and teach and not worry about all this," he says, gesturing around the pristine studio. "People want a nice clean room. They don't want a smelly, stinky mat. How do you do that if you don't have money? So having the balance and using the material for the right reasons is what we are doing," he says.

Given Finger's comments, it's legitimate to question the role of spirituality in the Yoga Works universe. Despite Wrubel's claim that people are looking for "balance and some center in their life," any talk of spirituality seems conspicuously absent at Yoga Works, at least at the studio I visited. "We definitely have detuned an overt spiritual message. We think it is enough for people to engage in the physical practice of yoga," Wrubel acknowledges. "We want to open the doors to people. We want them to begin from wherever they are in yoga and help guide them. But we don't want to create barriers from the very beginning either," Lichter adds. Which, of course, means that a Yoga Works class looks like just about every other yoga class in the Western world—a dressed-up aerobics routine. "It's fitness. That's certainly not our end goal, but we have to acknowledge that it's out there," Lichter concedes.

The buzzword at Yoga Works is not transcendence or enlightenment or even serenity. What Lichter and Wrubel strive for is *accessibility*. "We have presented a more accessible face to what has been a forty-thousand-year-old tradition to people. I think people are really open it," Wrubel says. But at what cost? Is accessibility coming at the expense of individuality, of the idiosyncrasies that often pull someone into a studio? I visit the Laughing Lotus yoga studio in Lower Manhattan to speak with cofounder and codirector Dana Flynn. Her class is a high-energy mash-up; Supertramp's "Logical Song" blasts from the speakers, students race through rigorous poses, sweat literally drips off the walls. All the while Flynn paces the room, exhorting, hectoring and enlightening her students. ("Yoga is a mirror for what's happening now!") It's a fast-paced, unique experience, a reflection of Flynn's hyperkinetic personality. "The classes here, the style of teaching, the over-the-top feeling in the place, the divine spark, if you will, it's so different here. Every place else looks the same. Go to L.A. Walk into every yoga center," Flynn says. "What's at the entrance? A Buddha and a waterfall. Every entrance at every yoga center is a little stone or a wooden Buddha…. They all look the same. They're all beige and dark wood and they have a Buddha and a waterfall." Her desire, she says, is to stand out. "It reflects our different personal sides. The way that I want to share yoga is even different from the way my partner shares yoga."[9]

Just over ten blocks from Laughing Lotus is Om Yoga, founded by Cyndi Lee. "Yoga is personal, totally personal; it's not generic," Lee says. "That's what keeps people coming back to a certain place. So, if it becomes less personal, it might not work."[10] Lee knows what she's talking about. She's been approached more than once to sell her business to a chain. "I've had those opportunities to actually join that vision or that business model. It's just not appealing to me right now," she says. Yet she remains realistic about what kind of squeeze a yoga chain like Yoga Works opening nearby would put on her. "That would be a drag, let's face it. I'm keeping my fingers crossed that they don't open right downstairs from me."

And that's the sad truth, says Trisha Lamb. No matter what the intentions of the owners might be, yoga chains will adversely affect the diversity of yoga experience. "Small, independent yoga studios will have a much more difficult time surviving because these large chain studios will be able to offer more kinds of classes, probably at a somewhat cheaper rate than the good little mom-and-pop yoga studio can afford to do. So, it will definitely have a long-range effect, particularly in large cities," she says. By this stage of our time together, Trisha's cherished impartiality is starting to crack. I ask her if the rise of yoga chains is a development that pleases or displeases her. "It makes me cry," she says, her eyes welling with tears.

There's no doubt that underneath all the passionately put arguments and well-rehearsed rhetoric, a vast ideological divide has developed over franchised yoga. This is a battle over what yoga is and what it should become, over new ideas and what Lichter calls yoga fundamentalism. And nerves are raw. "One of the things that we found most startling and distressing when we came into yoga is how quickly yogis can claim that other yogis aren't yogic. All of a sudden everyone's going, 'That's not yogic … she's not … he's not … they aren't.' So everyone's kind of squabbling," Lichter says. "Instead of coming together, they [yogis] are coming apart. That's scary stuff for us, so we certainly don't want to contribute to that."

Fuck Yoga

If one man has benefited from any bad vibes the yoga industry has given off it would be Barnaby Harris. You've got to admire a man like this, if only because he's figured out how to make a living doing something very simple. Barnaby sells yoga wear: T-shirts, mats, flip-flops and the like. But it's the not the gear itself that's caught on, it's Barnaby's message. Everything he sells is emblazoned with the simple slogan "Fuck Yoga." Another reason to admire him.

The Right Fit

"The first on-line sale came from two brothers in Bogotá, Colombia, and the second from a cheerleader in Grand Island, Nebraska. Since then we've filled in a lot of the map."

—Barnaby Harris, summarizing on his website
the exponential growth of his Fuck Yoga clothing line.

I first called Barnaby to see if he was interested in appearing in the documentary I'd been making. He said sure and invited me down to his cramped but cozy Lower Manhattan store one cold winter night. When I arrived the door was locked and the lights were out. I knocked. A disheveled, bleary-eyed figure emerged, hair askew, one shoe on, one shoe elsewhere. I had the distinct feeling I'd woken him up. (It was about 6 P.M.) It didn't seem to matter. Barnaby opened the door, I flicked on my camera and within seconds he had shrugged off his stupor and was talking a mile a minute. "Is there an alternative to this bullshit? I mean, everyone's marching around with a yoga mat and they think it's the goddamn Torah," he began. I asked Barnaby about the evolution of his impressively streamlined operation. He claimed the whole thing started by accident, the result of his now ex-wife's growing obsession with yoga. "I'd walk into the house and my wife was going to yoga. Yoga before dinner, yoga before this, yoga before that. I was like, 'fuck yoga.' " Inspired, Barnaby made her a T-shirt to that effect as a birthday gift. She refused to wear it, so he did—for thirty-nine days straight. "Next thing you know I was selling shirts in Johannesburg, Vienna, San Diego, Oregon, Bogotá. I think I probably sold close to a thousand shirts all over the world," he recalled expansively. "It's kind of the 'Shit Happens' of the new millennium."

Barnaby continued, unprompted. "The kicker is this. Here it is. Yoga has gone unopposed for thousands of years. Come on, already! I'm sure there was some sucker four thousand years ago standing in the back of some stone temple doing yoga with all those people thinking, 'What the fuck am I doing here?' but didn't speak up because he would have gotten his head cut off or his arms chopped off or incinerated or whatever they did."

Barnaby seemed busy, and I'd gotten plenty of material. But there was one last thing I wanted to ask him. He'd mentioned how difficult it was coming up with follow-up shirts to rival the pithy precision of "Fuck Yoga." But I'd been told he was on to something. It involved Sting, and I wondered if—"Fuck Sting. That is a brilliant shirt," Barnaby cut in. It was an idea he'd given much consideration but eventually rejected, for good reason, it turns out. "He's incorporated in the yoga shirt. 'Fuck Yoga' means 'Fuck Sting.' "

Although Sting is not the only name that comes to mind when people think "Fuck Yoga."

5

The Guru Who Laid
the Golden Egg

I have balls like atom bombs, two of them,
100 megatons each. Nobody fucks with me.
—BIKRAM CHOUDHURY, QUOTED IN PAUL KEEGAN,
"YOGIS BEHAVING BADLY," *BUSINESS 2.0*

If "McYoga" has become the catchall moniker for everything yoga traditionalists dislike about the industry, then Bikram Choudhury has become the Master of McYoga. Bikram, as he is almost universally known, has managed to find himself at the center of endless yoga hullabaloos. He's the millionaire yogi lording over an empire he defends with cutthroat legal precision; the bombastic showman determined to redefine yoga not as spirituality but as sport; the Hollywood hot-yoga guru whose roster of hotties and power players can overpower his message. (Acolytes have included Shirley MacLaine, Brooke Shields, John McEnroe, Madonna, Raquel Welch, Quincy Jones, Candice Bergen and basketball star Kareem Abdul-Jabbar.)

Wild assertions about Bikram are plentiful, but facts are a little harder to come by. He was (probably) born in 1946. He grew up on the mean streets of Kolkata, surrounded by poverty. He discovered yoga at age four, not atypical for a young Indian boy. His guru was the renowned and sought-after yogi Bishnu Ghosh, who ran the College of Physical Education in Kolkata and was the brother of

Paramahansa Yogananda, the influential guru who founded the Self-Realization Fellowship in the United States in the early twenties. Bikram was said to practice yoga four to six hours a day at Ghosh's college. At age thirteen Bikram won something called the National India Yoga Contest and remained undefeated for three years. This oft-repeated piece of Bikram lore is difficult to verify.

Choudhury then became a weightlifter, purportedly winning the similarly hard-to-verify All India Weight Lifting Competition in 1963, at age sixteen.[1] Many Bikram biographies also have him competing as a weightlifter in the 1964 Tokyo Olympics, although the official Olympic Games website has no record of him competing. His weightlifting career Bikram might have continued, too, if at age seventeen he hadn't allegedly dropped a 380-pound barbell on his knee. Told he would never walk again, Bikram turned again to his guru and teacher, Bishnu Ghosh. After six months of intensive yoga, Bikram has said, his knee was completely healed. Ghosh later asked his star pupil to start yoga schools in India and, after their success, to open a school in Japan. From there Guru Ghosh told Bikram to go west, young yogi. Another version of what brought Bikram west has Shirley MacLaine, who had studied with him in India, campaigning for her teacher to come to the United States. But the most colorful version involves none other than former American president Richard Nixon.

Among his many afflictions and idiosyncrasies, Nixon had since 1964 suffered from phlebitis, or deep-vein thrombosis, in his left leg. The condition had disabled him more than once, and in 1974 *Time* magazine reported on a particularly bad occurrence during an already tumultuous time in his life. "Less than three months after he was forced to resign the presidency, Nixon lay in critical condition in Long Beach Memorial Hospital Medical Center," the article said, with an inflammation that could "at any time cause a fatal blood clot to travel upward in the bloodstream through his heart to the lungs."[2]

In 1972, around the time of his historic visit to China, Nixon was in the South Pacific when the phlebitis flared up. This time he was lucky, it seems. Bikram Choudhury was on hand to administer his special hot yoga treatment. (*How* he came to be so close by has never been explained.) Soon Nixon was back on his feet. "He asked me

first thing, 'Sir, who are you? Are you an Indian black magician?' "
Choudhury recalled in a *60 Minutes* interview years later.[3]
Choudhury told Nixon he was a yogi, after which Nixon allegedly
gave Choudhury an open invitation to come and live in the United
States, complete with green card, in order to start yoga schools. (It's
the sort of amnesty for illegals that American conservatives could
never get away with nowadays.) Of course, there's not a shred of evidence to support the story. Even a representative from the Nixon
Library seemed baffled by my request for information about the
relationship, curtly replying via email, "We don't have any information regarding Mr. Choudhury and President Nixon."[4]

Accuracy and verifiability are not high on the list of qualities
Bikram loyalists value. Esak Garcia was introduced to Bikram Yoga
through his mother and older sister, who both teach it. In his junior
year of high school, Esak took his first yoga class with Bikram himself. He's since become Bikram's underling and close friend. "I would
like for all that to be true, that Richard Nixon sponsored him to
come to the United States; I would like for that to be true. But if it
is not true I still feel like I have faith in Bikram. I still have the same
love for him," Esak says. "Everyone likes to exaggerate. He speaks in
big absolutes and it's entertaining and I take it with a grain of salt."[5]

Bikram arrived in the United States, somehow or other, in 1973
and soon set up a studio in the Beverly Hills district of Los Angeles.
He must have been an anachronistic figure: Into an America still
bewitched by all things Eastern, onto streets paved with gold, had
been delivered this handsome, young, strong Indian man who was
(at that time) celibate, who didn't drink or smoke and who was by
all accounts shy to the point of it being debilitating. Good thing
Bikram's focus wasn't Hollywood. It was yoga, all the time, to the
exclusion of everything else. Legend has it he slept on his studio
floor. All he wanted was for people to attend his classes. "My school
was free. We don't think to charge money. For us, a yoga school is
like a temple. I had a little box, and people could put money in it.
Like a church," he told the *Los Angeles Times* in 2002.[6] It continued
that way until his devoted student Shirley MacLaine allegedly hired
him a manager and a security guard and told him to start making
some money. All the while Bikram was refining his now-famous hot

yoga technique of twenty-six poses and two breathing exercises, a formula as familiar to Bikram yogis as "two all-beef patties, special sauce, lettuce, cheese, pickles, onions on a sesame seed bun" became to hamburger fans. (And no, that's not the last time you'll hear McDonald's and Bikram being referred to in the same sentence.) Bikram Yoga (Bikram insists on a capital *B* and *Y*) is a series of twenty-six poses carefully culled from the eighty-four classical yoga postures, all performed in a room with the heat jacked up to somewhere near 105 degrees Fahrenheit (40 degrees Celsius). The heat, designed to help the muscles stretch, is what really makes the series unique—and so demanding. A Bikram class is ninety minutes of intense bending, stretching and sweating. Practitioners call it (affectionately) "Bikram's Torture Chamber." It's pure adrenalin, a physical endurance test, yoga without the bullshit, according to aficionados. So if it's meditation and enlightenment you want, you came to the wrong place.

It's Bikram that people usually have in mind when they talk about the "yoga business." Today Bikram Yoga is a worldwide phenomenon, a multimillion-dollar empire of over 1600 (by last count) studios catering to 50 million students, from Singapore to South Africa. Twenty-two Bikram studios are spread out across Japan, nearly forty across Canada. In Australia Bikram's eighteen studios eclipse the profile of any other yoga style, to the point where the words *yoga* and *Bikram* are almost synonymous.

What rankles so many people in the yoga world is that Bikram seems content to be perceived as a businessman first and a yogi second. In fact, he revels in his material success. Bikram claims not to know his personal worth but told Reuters in a 2008 interview that another magazine had estimated it at $3.5 billion.[7] And he's often seen tooling around Los Angeles in one of his fleet of classic cars, maybe the glittering white Rolls-Royce emblazoned with the vanity plate reading "Bikram," perhaps the Royal Daimler with a toilet inside that used to belong to Howard Hughes. Or maybe the black-cherry Phantom, which the Queen Mother used to tool around in. Or even the James Bond Aston Martin from the film *Thunderball.* "When I'm in India I do things like an Indian. When I'm in Japan, I'm a samurai. And when in Hollywood, I'm a playboy," Bikram told

---

A Worldwide Yoga Empire

Countries in which Bikram Yoga has studios:

Australia	Germany	Mexico
Austria	Hong Kong	Netherlands
Belgium	Hungary	New Zealand
Canada	India	Philippines
Chile	Indonesia	Singapore
China	Ireland	South Africa
Colombia	Israel	Spain
Costa Rica	Italy	Sweden
Czech Republic	Japan	Switzerland
England	Korea	Thailand
Finland	Malaysia	United Arab Emirates
France		

Reuters. "A yogi who has no attachment to material things lives in caves, lives for himself in the Himalayas. We had to come out of caves, go to ugly society and help the society."[8]

Journalist and yogi Andrew Vontz has written about Bikram for *FHM* magazine. "You have a lot of people complaining about a guy who's basically a classic entrepreneurial, up-by-the-boot-straps American success story," Vontz tells me. "Generally, Americans applaud these kinds of things."[9] (Vontz had never practiced Bikram Yoga before meeting Bikram but wants to now. "I would like my testicles to be atomic bombs," he says.)

Bikram's distinct personal style further blurs the line between shaman and showman. For formal occasions he usually favors one of his trademark silk suits, his long, thinning hair trailing down his back and usually topped with one of his multihued fedoras. The overall impression is of an Indian Al Capone, the Boss Hogg of Yoga, a bling version of the great sages of old. (Vontz likens the look to "*Thriller*-era Michael Jackson.") Bikram's typical teaching get-up is minimalist—and much more startling: a tiny black G-string Speedo, his hair imprisoned in an impossible-looking topknot. It's hard to believe this is the same shy boy of 1973. "He loves being 'The Bad Boy of Yoga,'" says Sandy McCauley, who runs three hot yoga studios with her husband, son and daughter in the Bay area of San Francisco.[10] McCauley was a student at Bikram's first-ever teacher training in Beverly Hills and remembers his frequent references to other yoga styles as "bullshit yoga." "I said, 'Bikram, are you sure you want to put out there into *Yoga Journal* and the public media that all other forms of yoga are bullshit? Is that the P.R. that we want to put out?' And his answer to me was, 'I can only tell the truth,'" McCauley recalls.

Ever the raconteur, Bikram is quick to grant interviews. And although he's never at a loss for contentious things to say about other yogis, he's just as willing to take criticism, and in fact seems oblivious to what people say about him. "Whatever people think of me, it doesn't matter. Those who know me, they love me and the world will do anything for me," Bikram told Reuters.[11] Although the many negative depictions may have turned Bikram into "a caricature of himself," according to Andrew Vontz, it certainly hasn't been bad for business. "Bikram quite correctly perceives that any publicity is good publicity. How many other yoga people can you name? How many gurus can the average American person reel off?" Vontz asks. "He has a brand name and he does what he can to promote himself. Good for him."

Bikram's handlers, however, must wince every time he opens his mouth to a reporter. Time after time they bemoan how misrepresented he is in the media, how different he is in person, how much of a softie he really is. It's true that describing Bikram on the printed page does not do him justice. On paper he comes across as an outsized megalomaniac, a slippery CEO in a Speedo. In real life he's much more of a loveable rogue. His energy is relentless and invigorating, his dedication to his students and craft is unwavering and the closeness between his wife, Rajashree, and their two children, Anurag and Luja, is touching and unself-conscious. (Bikram wed Rajashree in 1984, in a traditional Indian arranged marriage. She was a famed yogini in India, a five-time winner of the All India Yoga Championship, according to her biography.) But the best thing in Bikram's favor, if you ask me, is his sense of humor; he's quick, irreverent and puerile to the point of potty-mouthed. In person it's much easier to understand just how often and how firmly his tongue is planted in his cheek.

The Yogi Hunter

Bikram's sense of humor has gotten him a long way in the usually sanctimonious world of yoga. But it also masks a capricious and sometimes vindictive streak, which my brief relationship with him may be proof of. I began tracking developments in the yoga world as far back as June 2003, in preparation for the documentary that this book is based on. My first priority, given that he was the center of so much controversy in yoga, was to get Bikram on tape. My proposal was simple. I wanted to discuss the yoga industry and his place in it. I wanted to give him an opportunity to speak his side of any issue for as long as he wanted. Yet getting Bikram to sit down for my cameras became a four-year odyssey, earning me the nickname "The Yogi Hunter" among friends. Bikram and I had many short, friendly encounters over the period. Each time I would tell him what I was doing and try to cajole him into it. Each time he would nod and say, "yes, yes." Each time he'd tell me to speak to his people, leaving me confident that *this* time it would happen. I would shoot off more emails to these "people," who seemed to adjust job titles and responsibilities constantly. I went through five "representatives," each of whom could "guarantee" they'd get Bikram to cooperate.

Finally, in February 2006, toward the very end of shooting the film, after I'd shot a class he'd taught, Bikram consented to an interview. Caught a little off-guard, I hastily cobbled together a decent-looking interview setting in his office. Suddenly there was Bikram, framed in my viewfinder, resplendent in his Speedo and diamond-studded gold Rolex watch, topknot still in place, reclining against a tiger-print towel he had draped over the back of his oversized office chair. Before the interview began I once again explained what I was doing—a documentary about the yoga industry and his place in it. He was slightly taken aback at the mention of a documentary, as if (remarkably but perhaps not unsurprisingly) his people had never given him my proposal. He insisted I'd have to clear everything he said in the interview with his agent and that I "probably wouldn't be able to use it" in the final film. We decided to do the interview anyway; I wasn't about to let this opportunity slip by. And it went very well. We warmed to each other. He answered my difficult questions perfectly, provocatively and hilariously. I thought we had a great thing going.

Whatever goodwill I might have imagined had developed between us soon evaporated. The next day, as my crew was setting up the cameras to film the competition, one of Bikram's representatives strode over and demanded we stop shooting and leave the event. No reason or explanation was given. It was just over. After three and a half years of toeing the line, we were no longer welcome. Any further contact with Bikram would now have to be through his agent at "ICM," we were told. I sat down with Bikram and tried to figure out what had transpired between yesterday's sit-down and now. Maybe one of his people had gotten in his ear about me. But it was no use. He was adamant about my handing over the tapes, which I wouldn't do. That was the last contact I had with Bikram.

It's a familiar cycle with Bikram, I'm told. You begin on the outer circle and slowly work your way to the inner sanctum. Then there's some inevitable breach of trust, often unspoken or unspecified, and you're out of the circle completely. I've known a few people who've done these laps before, and they tell me it's just as easy to get back into Bikram's good graces. He'll suddenly call you up in the middle of the night, you'll find yourself at his next event and all will be forgotten, never to be spoken of again. If so, that's to his credit. But his handlers would be naive to expect anyone in the media or the culture beyond yoga to have the patience for such palaver. No wonder his public persona has become so cockeyed.

Bikram is an anomaly in yoga, a savvy, showy entrepreneur in an industry that eschews most outward displays of success. "It's a common denominator among many quasi-Socialist-type movements and spiritual movements, where you can't have anyone emerge as a capitalist figure, someone interested in making any money off it or someone with a very strong point of view. Because if any one person does those things, then it somehow brings down the community or the collective," says Andrew Vontz. Bikram, meanwhile, is quite pleased to stand out as what Vontz calls "a very aggressive capitalist." Nor does Bikram show any sign of slowing down or changing his ways. For many years he's been formulating a franchise plan, a logical extension, perhaps, of his rigorously conformist yoga style. "We expect to expand worldwide and have our yoga program and philosophy in every major city in the world," Bikram's Yoga College of India CEO Leslie LaPage told the *San Francisco Chronicle* in 2002.[12]

Under the franchise plan, studios from Kolkata to Kansas City would be the same. Physically identical, ideally with a mirror on every wall to compel students to concentrate on their outward form, and with carpet on the floor to aid traction. All studios would be strictly heated to no less than 105 degrees Fahrenheit. And every student would be guided through class with an identical ninety-minute dialogue, all doled out by Bikram-accredited teachers. That means all studio owners and teachers would require certification by Choudhury, a stamp of approval that doesn't come cheap. Students must cough up $6900 for the nine-week teacher training and $3900 for accommodation (two students per room), plus a few additional fees here and there. Then they must pay their way to the teacher-training facility in Acapulco, Mexico. If they become accredited, an outcome that is in no way guaranteed, they may open a franchise. At that point franchise owners would pay Choudhury a monthly fee based on the studio's gross monthly revenues.

In the nonconfrontational, life-affirming and self-empowering world of yoga, it's somehow considered indecorous to pass judgment on others. There is no good and bad, there is only different. This is a group of people, according to Vontz, "afraid of having negative reactions to things, or expressing negative emotions." Except when it comes to Bikram. Even Trisha Lamb has taken the gloves off, telling the *San Francisco Chronicle* in 2002 that Bikram's plan to build a franchise around a spiritual discipline is non-yogic and asserting, "Yoga is not hamburgers."[13] And although Bikram's systemized method for delivering more yoga to more people is not so different from the Yoga Works model, Yoga Works cofounder George Lichter distances himself from the Bikram method with vigor. "The McYoga is out there, and it's over there," he says. "That's what Bikram already represents. And that's a prepackaged form of yoga, where the script is the same, every word, every experience is the same." In contrast, Lichter explains, the Yoga Works model rejects conformity: "Every instructor is encouraged to put her or his soul and mind into the practice, so that there's no interest in standardizing." In the end, though, Lichter's assertions sound a lot like the squabbling he's accused other yogis of.

Andrew Vontz finds it easy to defend Bikram's franchise plan. "The macro effect … could very well be that thousands if not millions of more people do yoga. And maybe they will stumble onto the 'spiritual' side and they'll find some kind of soothing or psychological calm through doing it," he says. Besides, marriages of convenience are happening all the time between yoga principles and market forces. Vontz suggests that the people most outraged by Bikram's franchise plans are being willfully ignorant: "It's fascinating that so many westerners are misinformed about the true nature and history [of yoga]. What angers them is that their precious, misconstrued view of the history of India and yoga and all of these things that are 'other' and foreign to them are being brought back to them in a very McDonald's kind of form. They don't want their precious little thing treated that way. They want it to be something they continue to *not* understand and they can project anything they want onto it."

By early 2008 a ruinous court battle (detailed in later pages) seemed to have derailed Bikram's franchising plan. Never one to be underestimated, however, Bikram claims on his website that the plan is still "under development and will be made available to applicants as soon as possible."[14] Even if the plan never gets off the ground, yoga purists will still have reason to scorn him. Bikram is, after all, the executive producer and main player behind perhaps the biggest McYoga melee of all, the development of a competitive yoga scene.

Defensive Pose

The results were in. "Employing the brash style that first brought him to prominence, Sri Dhananjai Bikram won the fifth annual International Yogi Competition yesterday with a world-record point total of 873.6," read the article. Getting off to a fast start, Bikram vanquished his nearest competitor, two-time champion Sri Salil

"The Hammer" Gupta. "He attained total consciousness (TC) in just 2 minutes, 34 seconds, and set the tone for the rest of the meet by repeatedly shouting, 'I'm blissful! You blissful?! I'm blissful!' to the other yogis," the article continued.[15]

I fell off my chair laughing. Of course, this was the intended response. The article "Monk Gloats" was in the satirical newspaper *The Onion,* after all. But this tall tale about "un-Buddhalike" Bikram and a band of loutish yogis would soon become more prophetic. The story wasn't the parallel universe it seemed to be. It was a funhouse reflection of actual developments brewing in the yoga world, developments I'd soon find myself in the middle of. It wouldn't be the last time I'd fall off my chair laughing.

By early 2003 I'd been a practicing Bikram yogi for about four years. There I was in class one day, struggling to hold my standing bow pose, when the instructor dropped a bombshell. "Work hard on this one," she said casually. "Standing bow is part of the upcoming yoga championship." I sprang involuntarily out of my pose, literally thrown off balance by the phrase "yoga competition" but even more startled by the familiar ring it had. Then it hit me. The *Onion* article. After class I peppered the instructor with questions. What yoga competition? When yoga competition? *Why?* Armed with the few facts she could provide, I dashed home and immediately buried myself in research, my brain aflame with the zeal that can come only when a documentary filmmaker realizes that real life events have rendered satire obsolete. The first World Yoga Championship was coming up in just a few months. I had my next film. At first I didn't know what form the film would take. Initially, I thought it might make an interesting five-minute exercise, something odd to do between real gigs. (It was only later that I uncovered all the other yoga rifts and dilemmas that constitute the rest of the film.) The thing I *did* know was that I needed to get to that championship. Soon I was on a plane headed—where else? Los Angeles.

The Staples Center Arena in downtown Los Angeles is a world-class sports and entertainment arena that has hosted iconic performers such as U2, Paul McCartney, Madonna and the Rolling Stones. It's home to no fewer than five professional sports franchises. The center also has been home to the 2000 Democratic National Convention, seven Grammy Awards shows, the WTA Tour Championships, the 2004 NBA All-Star Game, countless championship boxing bouts and a ten-date, sold-out WWE run. At first glance the event unfolding at the Staples Convention Center this weekend, the first World Yoga Championship to be held in the United States, promises the metaphysical equivalent of a twelve-round WWE *SmackDown.* Bikram Choudhury and Deepak Chopra stand at the top of a long escalator, surveying the crowds that enter the main meeting hall. (Choudhury and Chopra are long-time friends.) A colossal LED display flashes announcements about upcoming events. Spectators and yogis trot to and fro amid an air of expectancy and excitement.

Bikram has pulled together a four-day yoga happening that he's called the Yoga Expo, a tradeshow featuring all manner of master classes, lectures and demonstrations. But there's little doubt that the yoga competition is the main attraction. The action unfolds in a large and typically lackluster boardroom jazzed up slightly for this event with a few statues and carefully arranged rugs. Well-wishers offer advice and snap pictures as competitors from across the globe, from Canada and Australia to India and Japan, psych and limber up. Mary Jarvis, a "yoga coach" from San Francisco, prowls around her charges with a watchful eye, offering advice and admonishment as they go through their warm-ups. "That! That! Everybody's doing that," she tells one yogi. "Move your knees to the mark. Good!" she says to another. "Those hands look sloppy," she tells a young yoga teacher from New York, reminding him to face out to the audience, presumably to better project his serenity. "Bright eyes, soft face," she says.

It's a little unclear exactly what *does* get you points here—serenity or suppleness. The official championship rules and regulations, which change slightly from competition to competition, are often a mix of stringent dictates ("Any stimulating drug or alcoholic beverage must not be used," "Female contestants must not be pregnant") and absurd vagueness (judges award points based on "dress," "style" and "proportion of the body"). The main criteria are usually the same, though: Participants must perform five compulsory yoga poses ("as derived from Patanjali") and two poses of their choice, all to be completed in three minutes. Each posture is judged on a scale of zero to ten, with judges paying attention to poise, grace, performance of postures and general appearance. Optional postures are judged on the degree of difficulty. Points are deducted for falls, imbalance, instability and exceeding the time limit. In other words, the judges aren't too concerned with your soul, it's your body they're interested in.

Participant Esak Garcia is perhaps the most articulate and passionate advocate for competitive yoga. Garcia believes the event *is* a measure of the soul in some way. "Yoga is a spiritual practice. It's a very personal, spiritual practice," Esak says. "When somebody is on stage, you can see their emotional state. You can see if they're nervous. You can see if their heart's beating fast. You can see if they are breathing hard, or if they're stressed. And I think that something about the human spirit *is* on display there."

Garcia is the perfect poster boy for competitive yoga. Soft-spoken, thoughtful and handsome, with a wide smile and long black hair, he's just the sort of telegenic pitchman the fledgling sport needs. With the right benefactor it could become a full-time gig, an idea he's given a lot of thought to. "It's only a matter of time before yoga athletes get sponsorships," Garcia tells me. His stance on corporate culture is convoluted, however. Garcia studied political science on a scholarship at Yale, receiving financial assistance from Mexican-American and Jewish foundations. (His father is Mexican, his mother Jewish.) At college he was a tireless campaigner against ruthless conglomerates and unchecked capitalism. As a member of Students for Corporate Responsibility, he even pressured Yale to divest from tobacco companies and other corporations that had low environmental and human rights standards. Now, with sponsorship on his mind, he's had to temper his attitudes toward some of those same corporations. "I am personally not a fan of the Nike Corporation, because when I was in college I was an activist and I studied and researched a lot of their practices in terms of how their workers are treated in other countries," he says. "But at the same time, if Nike wanted to give me money—I know they have a lot of money—and if they wanted to put that into promoting yoga I would accept that." He's quick to add that any such deal would have to include some kind of clause allowing him to criticize his sponsor. "Within each individual there are limits as to their 'commercialism,' what they're willing to do for how much money," he asserts.

Garcia spends much of his time traveling around the world demonstrating and teaching Bikram Yoga and preaching the gospel of competitive yoga. He meets many naysayers but takes them all in stride. "I feel very committed to the project," he says simply. Other competitors also recognize that the event rankles traditionalists. "I was actually still thinking about it until the day, if I was going to do it or not. But in the end, it just seemed like the right thing to do," says Jessica Murray, a Bikram Yoga instructor from New York. "I can't think of it as a competition at all. I'm a dancer, so for me, I just think of it as a performance, and that's how I manage," she says.[16]

"There is competition in yoga, whether you are willing to acknowledge it or not. People come here to class and they are comparing themselves to their neighbors; 'I'm more flexible than you, I'm stronger than you.' They compete for the teacher's attention," Esak contends. "To make it a positive thing, to say, 'Let's compete in yoga, this is an appropriate arena to compete in,' allows us to shape the competition into something that we are proud of. It gives us a means to compete and not betray our values," he adds.

That's not how the overwhelming majority of yogis see it. Most industry figures believe stripping the practice down to merely the physical poses misses the entire point of yoga. "If we enshrine the physical practice," says George Lichter, "we are condoning an understanding of yoga that falls far short of yoga's potential." Renowned teacher Rodney Yee calls competitive yoga an oxymoron and says that imposing a competitive structure onto yoga may have unintended and ugly results: "We're in a very competitive society already, so when you start putting those parameters on it again, you're going to get some nasty stuff." James Barkan, who was schooled in the Bikram method, calls the competition "sort of silly." "But at the same time, if they want to do it, I don't necessarily oppose it. I don't think it's blasphemous. Let them do it," he says. Trisha Lamb is more adamant, describing competition as the antithesis of yoga. "The teaching of yoga is to teach us that the duality that we are always stuck with, the 'me' versus 'you,' is not real. There is no 'me,' there is no 'you,' there is only our true nature," she says. "Participating in a competition, you are right there solidifying the 'I' am going to compete against 'you.' So that flies in the face of the core yogic teachings, for me."

To get beyond what Andrew Vontz calls "the politics of yoga," the rise of these yoga "athletes," as they prefer to be called, must be seen in perspective. In the West, yoga is primarily a physical pursuit, already stripped of its mind-soul associations. "To me, these people are certainly athletes. What we see them doing physically is a manifestation of the mastery of the *physical* practice of yoga," says Vontz. He adds that yoga competitions have a long history in India, where they are viewed as legitimate and popular events: "We have two worlds colliding, the East and the West.... It seems all the resistance is coming from the West, from people who are Johnny-come-lately yogis and yoginis, who don't really know that much about the history of yoga and are protesting something that, in fact, has a far more distant historical antecedent than their argument."

The reputed length of this history varies. Bikramites have told me yoga championships have been happening for everything from "many years" to "hundreds of years" to "thousands of years." And although these long and illustrious annals might be taken as gospel by many Bikram followers, the facts don't seem to support the assertions. "I don't think you can say there have been yoga championships for centuries, because there hasn't been *yoga* as we know it for centuries," says yogini and author Elizabeth Kadetsky, who studied yoga's murky history for her book *First There Is a Mountain: A Yoga Romance*. Kadetsky says the closest analogy history might offer are the Sanskrit competitions that date back to the tenth century. Competitors would try to outdo one another with increasingly complicated recitations of Sanskrit, South Asia's classical language, akin to Latin and Greek in ancient Europe. Sanskrit competitions are still held in schools today, largely as an attempt to revive that languishing tongue. But a historical *Hatha* yoga championship? "It's unverifiable," Kadetsky asserts.

According to my research, the oldest *verifiable* Hatha yoga championship, as Bikram's camp defines it, in which yogis actually compete against one another to perform physical poses, dates back to the late eighties. Additional filmed and anecdotal evidence exists of what *could* be competitive yoga dating back perhaps twenty years earlier than that.[17] But it's important to keep the context in mind. Bikram's people say championships "like these" have been going on for decades, yet the circumstances are so wildly different as to render any comparison almost worthless. Let's say hypothetically that a yoga championship happened in 1960 in India. Five decades ago India was a pious and conservative country. (That's true even of today's vastly transformed Indian culture, at least compared with the West.) Typical yogis of that time, the overwhelming majority of whom would have been men, were bound by rigid dictates about renunciation and modesty. Bikram's competitive yogis are primarily upper- and middle-class young men *and* women, whose scanty attire makes the average swimsuit look like full-body armor. Bikram's yoga championship takes place under klieg lights and surrounded by corporate branding in that most secular of temples, the sports arena. One can imagine the competitive yogis of old running for the exits—if they could get past that wall of merchandise in the Yoga Expo hall.

The past doesn't much matter to Esak Garcia. He's focused on today's events. His aim is not to beat other yogis but to beat his own personal best. "In that sense, the yogi competitor can ... not only use that powerful force of competition to realize his own or her own potential but to help each competitor to realize *their* own potential," he says. "We're just striving to be the best we can be and we're all doing it together."

Fair enough. Now, let's see who's going to win that gold cup.

We Are the Champions

The atmosphere inside the competition boardroom is heating up. Thirty or so competitors go through final preparations. Audience members, made up mostly of yoga students, teachers and competitors' friends and coworkers, take their seats and chatter among themselves. A string of elderly Indian gentlemen sit at a long table, sharpening pencils and conferring with Bikram. These are the judges. There seems to be some confusion as one of Bikram's staff bobs around, taking orders. "Seven milk, no sugar?" the young man

---

Rules of the Game

Excerpts from the Rules and Regulations for the International Yoga Asana Championships (available online at www.bikramyogasp.com/rules):

1. Each posture will be judged on a scale of 0 to 10 points.

2. If the performance is longer than 3 minutes the posture will be considered incomplete and disqualified.

3. Each posture is to be performed with stability and appropriate use of the time to finish the pose.

4. Contestants will be judged on the following criteria:
   - Walk
   - Movement
   - General appearance
   - Gracefulness
   - Performance of postures

The Judges will consider:

a) Performance regarding steadiness of the posture and execution of the pose.

b) Dress, style, and grace in asana execution.

---

asks. "With sugar, with sugar," a judge responds. "I'll bring sugar separate," the young man says, and dashes off.

The competitors have lined up behind the stage. Bikram leans into the microphone. The crowd falls quiet. "Welcome to first world championship of yoga," he says. The crowd applauds. "Thank you very much for coming. Let's officially start the competition." With that begins a procession of pliancy and sinuousness that borders on the bizarre, as one strikingly svelte and lissome young yogi and yogini after another take to the stage to work quietly through their postures. It's an absolutely excruciating affair to watch, even to a spectator like me, who's at least physically familiar with the Bikram Yoga poses. The competitors don't seem bothered in the least. Most of them manage to maintain a smile throughout, which will gain them points. They're like the chorus line in a big Broadway musical, a stable of entertainment workhorses who can run, jump, twist and split their way through two hours of exhausting stagecraft and still manage to sport wide, toothy, sweaty grins for the final curtain. (That shouldn't be surprising. In real life many of these competitors are professional dancers and actors.)

The aged Indian judges are doing an equally sturdy job in their role of critics. They sit at their table close to the stage, sipping their Starbucks and keeping poker faces. After each competitor leaves the stage they pick up their pencils in unison to take careful notes. Audience members also play their part, turning to one another after each performance to nod approvingly or shake their heads in dismay, an undulating display recognizing exemplars or deficiencies of yogic form, the subtleties of which are almost certainly lost on most outside observers.

After ten competitors go through the motions, a feeling of seen-one-seen-'em-all comes over me. I decide to check out the rest of the Yoga Expo, so wander off across the hall, past the signs for the Fashion Show and Mantra Girl, whoever she might be. I peruse the pamphlets for Maitreya Solar Crosses, Yoga in the Yucatan getaways, Yoga Birth classes and NEW YOGA FLOORING! I wander into the main vendor area. This is where the real action is, where accredited sellers hawk anything even remotely yogic or Eastern. I stroll past a dry-ice waterfall toward a man selling tiny bronze Indian figurines housed inside a tiny temple. I dawdle past a booth where I can experience "Energetic balancing," saunter past an opportunity to "Win, Win, Win Free Weekend Spa Retreat." I stop at the "yGuide Yoga Software" booth, where a young woman leads me through the software's "full-on practice tools." "All of the data is preloaded," she says. Across from her a robed woman sits atop a contraption consisting of ropes and pulleys that looks positively nineteenth century. This is SAM, the Spinal Analysis Machine. I decline the "Free Spinal Check!" Across the way a New Age artisan is selling paintings with a naked-angel-couples motif. I catch snippets of what she's saying to someone, something about "eternal" and "glistening wings" and "the light from the distance." Suddenly she grabs hold of me. After five minutes of her monologue I decide maybe a direct question is my way out and (regretfully) ask, "What was your inspiration?" Her answer has something to do with her resemblance to "a radio, tuning into different things. I select my stations!"

Eventually free, I escape toward the back of the hall, where a sweaty, long-haired, skinny white dude plays guitar while an intense black percussionist decked out in African garb bangs away fervently on a djembe drum. Neo-hippies bop about, grooving to the world beat in their flowing, spacey way. "Roll out the thunder!" the dude sings. A shirtless, muscular multiracial kid busts out some yoga moves as a girl of indeterminate age and ethnicity in green draw-string pants break-dances in front of him. "Into the ni-ight!" the singer continues.

I look for the exit. One wrong turn and I'm surrounded by a bunch of yogis in blazing red Bikram Yoga Expo T-shirts. This is the Bikram stall, and naturally all things Bikram are up for grabs. There's his *Bikram's Lounge* CD, on which he sings all the songs. Here's his *Beginning Yoga Class* book. Over there are a few huge laminated posters of Bikram sitting in lotus position on a tiger-skin rug. There's even a new compilation CD produced by Bikram, the *Yoga Expo Fashion Show Music Mix*. Now I need to leave. I'm nearly out when I stumble across the Mahatma Rice Mix booth, emblazoned with the rather muddled Mahatma logo, which looks to me like either a mystical Indian raj or a turbaned guru with a magic wand. The Mahatma staff is doling out free rice. A mom with two kids approaches. "Oh, our favorite," she says, taking several rice samples and passing them to her unimpressed progeny. She takes five pencils for the kids. They're free.

This is not a place for the cynical.

Days Two and Three of the expo blend together in a whirlwind of yoga competition and commerce. Poses are struck, goods are exchanged, repeat. An event on Day Three stands out, however: an attempt by Bikram to break the Guinness World Record for the largest yoga class ever held. By Bikram's count at least thirteen hundred people have jammed into one of the convention center's enormous inside arenas, although that's not enough people to break the record. (Bikram claims the room can't hold more people because of safety restrictions.) Anyway, the world record bid is really just an opportunity for Bikram to deliver a lecture to a large group, something he relishes doing. He prowls across the stage in his tiny black Speedo and headset, scolding the crowd for growing up in the West, the "wrong place," and therefore having no real moral compass. Then he offers the possibility of redemption. "You have one hope. I don't want you to die in the wrong place. That's why, right now, you are at the right place. Welcome to Bikram's Torture Chamber!" And with that familiar refrain a good portion of the crowd erupts in applause. This is the Bikram his followers know and love, the master of rodomontade, the cartoonish braggart who just so happens to have developed a system of physical and mental rejuvenation they swear by. "That's why I am the smartest man in the world you ever met in your entire life. I make a package," he continues. "The best-selling product in the world of all time, imported from India. Bikram Torture Chamber. Twenty-six postures, two breathing exercises. It works!" The crowd erupts again.

After just two more hours of Bikram berating, belittling and bewitching us, the class begins. It's a diverse crowd. Among the usual throng of twentysomethings is an older Indian gentleman in traditional clothing. Next to him, a fiftysomething woman who looks as if she came straight from the Botox chair. Nearby, a middle-aged man executes his poses in a suit and tie. There's a fair smattering of children as well, showing admirable and mature focus. From his perch on stage Bikram pushes all of us to go farther, delivering the dialogue that has become so familiar and so comforting to Bikram acolytes worldwide: "Full lungs. All the way up. Exhale out ... Lean back, back, back, way back, all the way back." And so on.

Day Four of the expo culminates in the moment most of us are here for, the yoga competition awards ceremony. Having been through various qualifying and elimination rituals, all the participants are now gathered on stage, waiting for the judges to tabulate their results. A man busily polishes a shimmering gold trophy as a mob of local media types lightly jostle one another to get the best cutaway.

Then Bikram addresses the crowd. His comments are aimed squarely at those who dare to question his competitive yoga push, who decry the event as nothing more than folly, an elaborate PR move designed to garner attention. "You are competing with yourself," Bikram says, repeating once more the motto that has become so familiar over the past few days. "So any idiot ask you how yoga can be competition, you better go back home and tell them, no, we didn't compete in America, Germany, Japan, India. We compete our body, mind, spirit to improve it in highest level in cosmic consciousness. That's it," he declares.

It's the moment we've all been waiting for, to see who's earned a two-week trip to the city of their choice, $3000 cash and that grandiose gold trophy. "First-place winner," the announcer intones, "goes to Lesli Christiansen!" A perky blond Bikram instructor and hairstylist from San Diego steps forward. Bikram places the gold medal around her neck. She breaks out in tears. Flashbulbs pop as the other competitors whoop and cheer excitedly. It takes more than a few minutes for the fuss to die down. Then I pull Lesli aside for an interview. She says her friends and family were supportive, although they were initially skeptical about mixing yoga and competition. "But they definitely mix together, because you're competing with yourself, with your mind and your body and your soul," she tells me. I ask what her strategy was going into the event. "My main actual goal was to be competing with myself, to show at least one part of my soul to the judges; that's how I knew that I would be a winner," she says.[18] I'm tempted to ask her if she's seen the famous Monty Python sketch in which a professional wrestler competes against himself in a five-round contest. He wins, and goes on to meet himself in the final. But I'm not sure she'd get the joke.

The Thrill of Victory

The championship is almost over when an offhand comment catches my attention. One of the judges rises to thank Bikram, and in so doing casually encapsulates the ultimate goal of the competitive yoga circuit. "I'm confident that this day will come, when yoga is included in the Olympic Games," he says.

Wait ... the *Olympics*? Like Jesse Owens Olympics? Like decathlon, javelin, long-jump Olympics? Apparently. Since at least 2003 the Bikram organization has been lobbying the International Olympic Committee to include yoga as an exhibition sport. "If gymnastics can be in the Olympics, why can't yoga be in the Olympics?" Bikram's wife, Rajashree, asks me during an indignant interview. "Gymnastics has scores. You have to complete this much bending, or jumping or things like that. Yoga also has a perfection," she says.[19] Trisha Lamb counters this by asking, "*Is* there a way to reach the perfection of the pose? What's perfect for me is not what's perfect for you. There is a sense that bodies look aesthetically pleasing to a group of judges. You could say that. But is that yoga? Is that in line with the purpose of yoga?" Lamb's tart response is typical of the derision the concept of Olympic yoga provokes. "There always has to be a winner in every Olympic event I've ever seen," says George Lichter. "And I don't see how you can deem someone has reached enlightenment faster than someone in lane three. It seems almost comedic."

Bikram's stated reason for wanting yoga included in the Olympics is to increase its popularity. The problem, says Andrew Vontz, is that one thing does not guarantee the other. "Look at the Olympics and some of the events that have made it into the Olympics, like the skeleton, which is a face-first luge on a bobsled track, or rhythmic gymnastics, which involves twirling around things on the end of sticks. Inclusion in the Olympics does not necessarily mean that a sport's going to become more popular or more people will participate in it," he says. He also questions what competitors will get out of it. "What would be the benefit of having an Olympic gold medal [for yoga]? Would you have a lucrative lululemon contract? Winning the world championship gets you a gift certificate to go to teacher training with Bikram?"

There's another hurdle to Bikram's Olympics bid. Although derived from the eighty-four classical yoga postures, the poses that Bikram Yoga competitors perform all come from the Bikram series. While an Iyengar yogi or Vinyasa practitioner would recognize the pose, he or she would be used to performing it quite differently. "There was an article in the *Yoga Journal* a couple of years ago about triangle pose done six different ways by six different major schools," says Rodney Yee. "Ashtanga yogis put their hands behind their heads. Some people take short strides. Some people take long strides." In the absence of a valid way of judging one yoga style against another, Bikram instead seems to be saying that *all* yoga competitions should be judged by his standards. There's one advantage to that: "At least you know what you're getting judged by. You have to look like Bikram!" Yee says with a chuckle. Then there's the fact that only one group of yogis has expressed any desire to see yoga become an Olympic event. "It's only the Bikram world that's into it. The rest of the world turns their nose to it," James Barkan says simply.

Despite all this, there's a sense among some yoga industry leaders that yoga *will* eventually become an Olympic sport. "It will probably happen," says Lamb. "But for me, it will be another form of gymnastics, it won't be yoga," Yoga Works cofounder Rob Wrubel offers a slightly warmer embrace. "If it shows up in the Olympics and that's someone's view of doing yoga, so be it," he says. Barkan just shrugs. "Baseball is in the Olympics and it's like, nobody really cares."

Convincing the Olympic committee to accept yoga as a new sport will be no small feat. It must first be proven that the "sport" in question is practiced in at least seventy-five countries over four continents. Then an international federation to govern yoga must be set up for the International Olympic Committee to recognize the sport. Finally, that federation must file an application for yoga to become a demonstration sport at the Olympics, then eventually a recognized Olympic sport. It's not clear whether the Bikram organization has filed the necessary paperwork. We know yoga wasn't part of the 2008 Beijing Games—despite Bikram's assertion to me three years earlier that China would host the "first Olympic trial, no question about it." The Bikramites belief in their leader remains unshakeable, however. "Bikram and Rajashree are very committed to and dedicated to getting yoga, or this form of competition, into the Olympics, and I believe that one day they will do that," says Satya, a devoted Bikram yogi. "I believe that in a very short time yoga will be in the Olympics," says Jeff Renfro, a studio owner and long-time friend of Bikram's. "If it's something that Bikram wants," one competitor tells me, "I would definitely back it and support it."

6

Karma Police

The word "yoga" has been vulgarized and does not
mean anything now.
—SWAMI RAMA, *PATH OF FIRE AND LIGHT:*
ADVANCED PRACTICES OF YOGA

For a great percentage of the world's population, daily life is endless hardship. Much of humanity lives with suffocating poverty, famine, political insecurity and ethnic warfare, conflicts that seem endless, insufferable and unsolvable. Some of this turbulence touches us in the West. Pictures on our TV and computer screens show us grief and give us pause. Commuters feel it at the gas pump. Mothers mourn sons and daughters who die fighting hard to fathom wars in far-off places. But many of us remain largely immune to this sort of misery. And no wonder. The Western lifestyle, no matter where it's being lived, offers a wealth of tawdry distractions: sports superstars who fall hard from undeserved grace, politicians with their pants down and their hands in the cookie jar, endless online videos of infantile celebrities caught in flagrante delicto. And if the great problems of the world or the pile of muck in our own backyards do get to be too much, we have a way out. We go to yoga.

Yoga has long been sold as an escape from daily life, a departure from the tawdry, depressing, mundane and malicious. That's why thirty years ago people were heading en masse for the ashrams.

People such as Dan Shaw, who went there as an escape from the emptiness of his life. "It was exciting and alluring. And I started to feel happier and more purposeful," he says.[1] Fifteen years ago, teacher training was the yoga escape du jour. That lawyer friend who was also into yoga would suddenly disappear for a few weeks. (India? Hawaii? Vermont?) When he returned it was with "certification" and a promising new career ahead of him. The current vogue is the yoga "getaway." Websites promote four-day weekend tours to far-flung places that offer "deep immersion" in yoga and promise to "enhance one's life, health and relationships." It's basically a weekend on the beach, with the option of a yoga class in the morning.

There's a troubling pattern here. It seems yogis are no longer making the long-term commitment to yoga that they used to. Could the bloom be off the rose? With so much going so apparently awry in the yoga world, has the claim of yoga as an escape from the grubbiness of real life lost the validity it once had? Yoga's history in the West has come to be seen as a wayward and often bawdy affair, a saga rife with power plays, outsized egos and sexual shenanigans. And there's no end of stories to corroborate this characterization. In 2002 a former instructor at Rodney Yee's yoga studio in California filed suit against Yee and his then-wife for breach of conduct. The woman claimed her lease had been terminated in retaliation for confronting Yee about his alleged extramarital affairs with his students. In 1997 a jury found Swami Rama, the spiritual leader of the Himalayan Institute in Pennsylvania, guilty of sexual misconduct after a woman claimed to have been sexually assaulted by him. The woman, nineteen years old at the time of the abuse, was awarded $275,000 in compensatory damages and $1.6 million in punitive damages. A year earlier the Ananda Church of Self-Realization was ordered by a California court to pay at least $625,000 to a former member who claimed to have been sexually exploited and defrauded by both the church's founder and a married senior church minister. And in 1994 Amrit Desai, founder and leader of the Kripalu Center for Yoga and Health, one of North America's largest holistic health centers, resigned after admitting he'd had affairs with three female followers—in flagrant violation of his own teaching of celibacy.

All these high jinks in less than ten years, and that's only in the United States. Then there are the constant flare-ups that revolve around yoga's big-business gurus, the fear that they've commercialized the practice beyond recognition, making dollars more important than dharma. It all raises the question, Shouldn't we expect more of our gurus? If we can't expect our so-called spiritual teachers to lead by example, whom can we trust? Is it time to call the karma police? In 2004 *Yoga Journal* kicked off a wave of hand-wringing with an article titled "Ethical Dilemma." The article envisioned the need for a Yoga Hall of Shame to house all the yogis who were guilty of "physical negligence, fraud, embezzlement, and ruthless business practices."[2] What had been a whisper among yogis for an enforceable, industry-wide yoga code of ethics became a full-throated cry. And the industry is taking notice.

Sounding more like a band of do-gooding superyogis, the Yoga Alliance is an American trade organization formed to "lead the yoga community, set standards, foster integrity, provide resources, and uphold the teachings of yoga," according to the group's mission statement. Like many yoga organizations, the Yoga Alliance already enforces a code of ethics. And, like many organizations, it has guidelines that focus mainly on the delicate nature of the teacher-student relationship, where the overwhelming majority of ethical lapses seem to germinate. Accordingly, the Yoga Alliance code of conduct asks that teachers "respect the rights, dignity, and privacy of all students" and "avoid words and actions that constitute sexual harassment," among other stipulations.[3] The California Yoga Teachers Association became the first American yoga organization to enforce its own code of conduct in the early nineties, and its dictates remain perhaps the most stringent in the industry. Recognizing that "the teacher-student relationship involves a power imbalance," the document requests that teachers "show sensitive regard for the moral, social and religious standards of students" and understand that "all forms of sexual behavior or harassment with students are unethical, even when a student invites or consents to such behavior or involvement."[4] The Kripalu Yoga Teachers Association guidelines require that teachers "never exploit the vulnerability of a student for personal gain or gratification."[5] The International Kundalini Yoga

Teachers Association, the training arm of 3HO founder Yogi Bhajan's empire, has an exhaustive code of professional standards that declares: "All forms of sexual involvement are unethical."[6]

Ethical reform of yoga is an issue worldwide, although outside the American industry the requirements are usually more forgiving. The code of ethics devised by the Iyengar Association of Canada, the country's governing body for Iyengar yoga, doesn't forbid intimate relationships between teacher and student. But if the student-teacher relationship has been "compromised by the existence of an intimate relationship," teachers are asked to "assist the student in finding another Iyengar yoga teacher if possible."[7] The British Wheel of Yoga, which bills itself as the governing body for yoga in the United Kingdom, has a "code of ethical practice" that doesn't expressly forbid anything, asking instead that teachers "encourage and guide students to accept responsibility for their own behaviour and practice."[8] The International Yoga Teachers Association of Australia, founded in 1967, asks that each signatory "teach with goodwill and respect for all."[9]

With all these codes, statements and guidelines, you'd expect the yoga world to be a well-regulated, wholesome arena. Not so, and for two reasons. First, there's no uniformity among these standards of conduct, so what goes for one style is verboten in another. How is the yoga student or teacher expected to keep up? Second, there's no all-encompassing national, let alone international, body governing the many yoga styles, so there's almost no enforcement of any of these rules. (This is the yoga world, after all.) Even within each style there is very little apparent enforcement. Only one of the ethical guidelines cited above offers any clue in its code of ethics about what will happen if the codes are broken. (The Australian-based International Yoga Teachers Association says an offending member "may have membership of this Association suspended or revoked.") In other words, most of these guidelines are toothless. "Voluntary" is how Judith Lasater, president of the California Yoga Teachers Association and a guiding force in creating that association's code of ethics, describes them. That might be for the best, from a legal standpoint anyway. A code of conduct signed by a teacher offers no legal guarantee that the teacher will act accordingly. But if an organization legally requires signatories to abide by its rules, then that organization may also be legally responsible if the teacher breaches those rules.

There are more hurdles to ethical reform. The role yoga teachers play in our society is very difficult to define. A teacher may take on many roles, depending on the class and students. One student's therapist is another student's fitness guru. One yogi's holistic healer is another yogi's spiritual guide. And the role the teacher plays may not even be of his or her own choosing. The culture is hungry for authenticity. We're eager for people to look up to, quick to imbue our teachers with qualities they may not have. As the US-based Kripalu Yoga Teachers Association code of ethics suggestively states, "Some students may idealize us or project that we are wiser or more evolved than they are." It's what *Yoga Journal* calls "the pedestal problem." Suddenly every teacher is considered a guru, whether they like it or not. "The word *guru* to me does not just mean 'teacher.' It's a much more serious word. It comes from a tradition where there's a real, not just spiritual, but real life-counseling situation taking place," says Rodney Yee. "*Guru* is a dangerous term, really."

These appointed-by-default gurus are then often saddled with unrealistic expectations they feel obligated to meet. "As teachers we are given a certain level of stature in people's eyes and made special in people's eyes. I think there is a responsibility, definitely, to uphold that healthy boundary between teacher and student," says Power yoga guru Baron Baptiste. But the idolatry aimed at teachers makes it even easier for them to succumb to the temptations of sexual, emotional and even financial control—a mystical vicious circle. Even Baptiste alludes to having gotten caught up. "A lot of teachers are kids in a candy store. I got that out of my system early," he told *People* magazine in 2003.[10]

To the already complicated matter of defining the yoga teacher's role you can add the fact that not all yoga styles emphasize the same values or encourage the same behavior. "It's hard to enforce a universal code when there are all these different camps and different styles," explains James Barkan, owner and director of the Barkan Method yoga school. "To say, 'Okay, now we have to enforce a new code of ethics,' it's almost a fascist implication." Barkan suggests yoga could do with a few less rules. "There's a lot of dogma in the yoga world. And I try to stay away from that," he says. Others question the intrusiveness of proposed reforms. Baron Baptiste concedes that blanket reform may be necessary. "If we need a moral code out there and ethics because we've lost our way as a yoga community, if we need it, then fine," he says. But he's quick to point out it's not something *he* requires: "I don't need a code of ethics, personally, because I already have ethics. I don't need a moral code, because I already have my own moral code." It's no wonder ethics reform has been a long time coming. "It's like herding cats," Judith Lasater told *Yoga Journal* in 1999, "to get all of these yoga groups together on professional standards."[11]

Yama Drama

Traditional yogis have a simple solution to the knotty ethical problems of present-day yoga. Let the practice provide the answer, they say, referring specifically to the eight-limbed path of yoga. Defined (probably) by the sage Patanjali (very) approximately 2000 years ago in the Yoga Sutras, the eight-limbed path is now widely regarded as the foundation of modern yoga. Called *Ashtanga* in Sanskrit (from *ashta*, meaning "eight," and *anga*, meaning "limb," each Ashtanga "limb" is preparation for the following step, with the first two limbs forming the ethical foundation on which yoga should be practiced. The first limb is the *yamas*, five restraints on behavior that every yogi must strive to uphold. The second limb is the *niyamas*, five observances covering matters such as cleanliness, discipline and austerity. Then comes *asana*, the discipline of the body; and *pranayama*, the control of breath. Next is *pratyahara*, the withdrawal of the senses; *dharana*, focused and external concentration; and *dhyana*, steadfast meditation. The eighth limb is the money shot, *samadhi*, liberation, complete control over the functions and distractions of consciousness.

Despite that the eight-limbed path is the backbone of the majority of modern yoga lineages, the sad truth is that most present-day yogis wouldn't know their ashtanga from their asana. "Yoga traditionally is based on moral disciplines and self-restraints," says Trisha Lamb. "We like to skip over that part in America." Most of us come to yoga for a physical workout and usually dive right in at the third step, asana, plunging straight into handstands and backbends without even knowing about the preceding two steps or the ethical base they provide. "You didn't start practicing asana—or posture—or pranayama—breath control—until you had a good moral foundation. That's not uppermost in the minds of most Americans," Lamb says.

A few yogis may decide after some months to go deeper with their practice. That's usually when they go winding, incorrectly, back *down* the eight-limb path to discover niyamas, the observances. While that may hold their interest for a while, it's on the first rung of the ladder, the yamas, where they really should be focused. These restraints (the word *yama* means "restraint," "abstention" or "self-discipline" in Sanskrit) have come to be seen as the bedrock of yoga philosophy, what Patanjali called the "great vow" of yoga. The first yama, *ahimsa,* counsels us to restrain against violence in thought, word and deed. The second yama is *satya,* to abstain from dishonesty in word and thought. The third yama, *asteya,* means noncovetousness, eliminating any desire for anything that is not rightfully yours. The fourth yama is *brahmacharya,* which means self-control, especially in sensual matters. The last yama is *aparigraha,* nonpossessiveness, abstaining from possessiveness, greed and selfishness.

"If you look at all the major spiritual traditions, they've all discovered some hard-and-fast rules that, if you disobey them, you kind of get off track," says Lamb. The yamas are no different. "If you follow them, everything unfolds very beautifully and with integrity," she says.

The yamas are further evidence of yoga's boundless ability to be all things to all people. These simple dictates are the closest thing to a religious creed that yoga has to offer. In fact, they're often referred to as the "Thou Shalt Nots" of yoga: Thou Shalt Not Harm, Thou Shalt Not Lie, Thou Shalt Not Steal, Thou Shalt Not Lust and Thou Shalt Not Be Greedy. Drawing on the yamas can reinforce yoga's air of religiosity. At the same time, and unlike the majority of established religions that assume familiarity with particular tenets, the practice of yoga does not require participants to believe in, adhere to

The Backbone of Yoga

According to Patanjali's eight-limbed path, considered the foundation of most modern yoga, each stage is preparation for the subsequent stage.

1. Yama

   The first limb, yama, deals with our ethical standards and sense of integrity. There are five yamas:
   - Ahimsa: nonviolence
   - Satya: truthfulness
   - Asteya: nonstealing
   - Brahmacharya: abstinence
   - Aparigraha: noncovetousness

2. Niyama

   The second limb, Niyama, has to do with self-discipline and spiritual observances. The five niyamas are
   - Saucha: cleanliness
   - Samtosa: contentment
   - Tapas: spiritual austerities
   - Svadhyaya: study scripture and self
   - Isvara pranidhana: surrender to God

3. Asana

   The third limb represents the physical postures practiced in yoga. Practicing asanas develops the yogi's discipline and concentration, which are necessary for meditation.

4. Pranayama

   The fourth limb is the control of breath, designed to gain mastery over the respiratory process while recognizing the connection between the breath, the mind, and the emotions.

5. Pratyahara

   The fifth limb means withdrawal, the conscious effort to draw our awareness away from the external world and outside stimuli.

(continued)

6. Dharana
   Dharana means concentration, learning how to slow down the thinking process by concentrating on, for example, a specific energetic center in the body or the silent repetition of a sound.

7. Dhyana
   The seventh limb is meditation, the uninterrupted flow of concentration and a state of awareness without focus.

8. Samadhi
   The eighth and final stage is a state of ecstasy, at which point the yogi transcends the Self altogether and realizes a profound connection to the Divine and all living things.

or even know about the yamas in order to be involved. Thus, the practice can also remain secular. This duality has contributed to a religion-lite quality that has allowed yoga to thrive in secular and religious societies alike. Take Canada and the United States as examples. In the fifties, almost seven out of ten Canadians attended weekly religious service. In just half a century that number had dropped to just two out of ten, partly because of increased immigration, as well as multiculturalism, globalization and sexual liberation. In the United States during the same fifty years, the percentage of regular religious attendance climbed steadily to its current level of roughly 35 percent of the population. Religion's role in the Canadian public square is limited; no Pledge of Allegiance in school, no "In God We Trust" on the currency. In contrast, American life is steeped in public displays of religion. Yet both countries have enthusiastically embraced and absorbed yoga into their culture.

That doesn't mean the relationship between church and studio is always cozy. Every few months brings news of some predictable flare-up between yoga and established religion, usually some nonsensical sect of fundamentalist Christianity. In January 2007

Christian parents in British Columbia were outraged that a school program to fight childhood obesity was incorporating yoga. The parents considered yoga a competing religion and didn't want their children exposed to it during class time, despite assurances from the school that yoga was being taught only as exercise and that children could opt out if they wanted to. For local rancher Audrey Cummings there was a larger concern at hand. "There's God and there's the devil, and the devil's not a gentleman. If you give him any kind of an opening, he will take that," she said.[12]

An April 2005 article posted on Christianity Today's website titled "The Truth about Yoga" warns people about the "spiritual pitfalls" of the practice. "Christian speaker/author Laurette Willis tells everyone she meets about the dangers of yoga," the article states. Willis cautions against the openness of mind that yogis seek. "If there's nothing in your mind, you're open to all kinds of deception. After coming to Christ, I wondered who—or what—came into my body when I 'stepped out,'" she is quoted as saying. (Christ didn't leave much room, evidently.) Luckily, Willis has a solution for yoga-starved disciples of Jesus: PraiseMoves, a gospel-infused fitness regimen she created that she calls "a Christian alternative to yoga."[13]

It should also be abundantly clear by now that yoga isn't the spiritual workout it once was. According to Stefanie Syman, author of *Practice: A History of Yoga in America*, as early as the fifties and sixties, yoga pioneers such as Indra Devi and Richard Hittleman were uncoupling yoga from its Hindu roots. "They talk a lot about the psychological dimension of yoga and they play down the spiritual, transformative part," she says. "No more rebirths, because that's not a part of the Judeo-Christian conception of the world." Now, with the line between workout and worship so thoroughly blurred, the faithful are taking yoga back—only this time it's the Christian faithful. With little apparent regard for yoga's long and storied links to the ancient Eastern faiths, "Christian yoga teachers" (naturally, they have formed a national association) are now retooling yoga entirely by simply fusing it with their beliefs. The result is a crudely grafted hybrid of detuned Hinduism, vestigial paganism and heavy-handed Christian proselytizing. In 2001 Susan Bordenkircher developed Outstretched in Worship, an instructional DVD series that combines yoga with her own Christian faith. When other yogis might be meditating, Bordenkircher's charges are citing Bible verse. "We're going to use the scripture today from Psalms 46," she says at the beginning of one DVD. "Just be still and know that He is God." Gone is sun salutation, the series of poses familiar to yogis the world over that honors the Hindu sun god. In its place is "Son" salutation, a shout-out to Jesus. Although it's not entirely clear which Jesus we're talking about. It's hard to imagine the strapping, bling-sporting Jesus of the prosperity gospel bothering with this stuff. And the downtrodden and bedraggled Jesus who seems to spend equal time shepherding the poor and scoring points for political candidates surely couldn't find the time. Only an entirely new kind of Jesus, a flexible, latte-sipping, metrosexual Jesus could be this unafraid of the yoga mat.

You can see yoga purists bursting at the seams over this sort of absurdity, battling with their yogic teaching of withholding judgment. On one hand, they insist, yoga cannot be unmoored from its Hindu roots and made an addendum to some unrelated faith system. "Yoga *is* Hinduism," says Subhas Tiwari, professor of yoga philosophy and meditation at the Hindu University of America in Florida.[14] (Even Laurette Willis, the creator of PraiseMoves, agrees with this sentiment. " 'Christian yoga' is an oxymoron," she declares.) On the other hand, purists want yoga to be open to people of all faiths to interpret as they wish, as a sort of universal, um … religion. It's a real bind. Should purists preach their own form of Hindu-centric yoga fundamentalism or open the gates to a Christian takeover? (They needn't worry about the Catholics, at least. A papal decree has taken care of them. A 1989 document issued by the Vatican and signed by then-cardinal Joseph Ratzinger, now Pope Benedict XVI, says Eastern traditions such as yoga "can degenerate into a cult of the body" and warns Catholics against mistaking yoga's "pleasing sensations" for "spiritual well-being.")[15]

All this seems ample proof of the old adage that spiritualism unites but religion divides. "We've always had religion in the West, but religion is different from spirituality," says Trisha Lamb with a

Rome versus Om

The 1989 document from Cardinal Joseph Ratzinger warning Christians about the spiritual dangers of Eastern meditation was a concerted response by the Church to the pull of Eastern religious practices. According to the twenty-three-page decree, the symbolism and body postures used in these practices can "become an idol and thus an obstacle to the raising up of the spirit of God." Giving significance to the sense of well-being brought on by meditation may also produce "a kind of mental schizophrenia which could also lead to psychic disturbance and, at times, to moral deviations," the document states.

Dr. Timothy Shriver, chairman of the Special Olympics and a lifelong Catholic, offered up a spirited defense of yoga in a 2008 column written just a week before Ratzinger's first tour of the United States as Pope. "The explosion of self-help books, spiritual guides, and Eastern religious practices are all indications that we are becoming a nation of seekers, less interested in the teachings of religions and more in the experiences of the spirit," Shriver wrote. "The cerebral theologian needs to interrupt his schedule, put on sweat clothes, and drop in on a yoga class when he's in town ... He'd find growing numbers of Americans who have turned to the ancient Hindu practice for both physical and spiritual centering."[16]

For whatever reason, Ratzinger was unable to take Shriver up on his Papal Yoga Challenge.

grin. The irony, of course, is that this whole fracas obscures the fact that yoga can benefit everyone. "Its [yoga's] purpose is never to convert you. It's to help you. It's to help you in whatever your religious orientation is," Lamb says.

All this talk of morals and purity and interpretation make questions about the ethical dimension of yoga all the more relevant. What role should the yamas play in the modern yoga scene? Is it too much to ask yoga industry leaders to adhere to these few basic rules? Or is that taking the slippery path to fundamentalism? Would abiding by the yamas solve the ethical problems so rampant in the industry? Is it realistic or even beneficial to expect yogis to stick to an almost impossibly high moral standard, even if it is intrinsic to a traditional definition of the practice? As Jivamukti's David Life told *Yoga Journal* when interviewed for the "Ethical Dilemma" article, "It doesn't do much good to recite something from 1000 B.C. and expect it to be relevant, unless you make it so."

According to Lamb, expecting yoga teachers, let alone students, to adhere to some ancient and arguably arbitrary morality goes against the nature of the average westerner. "We like to do what we like to do. Morality is relative. I have my morality. You have yours. There's no hard and fast rules," she says. Besides, few yogis even know, much less care, about the sutras, the yamas or any other ethical dimension of yoga. (One Bikram yogi I spoke to went on at length about the "yoga sutras of Bengali" without being able to list any. "I'm blanking right now because I can't really remember all the names. But it all comes from that. The ancient yogis that do all these postures. Therapeutically." Uh-huh.)

Author and yoga historian Elizabeth Kadetsky argues that it's folly to place so much emphasis on such a small aspect of yoga philosophy. "This yoga subculture has latched on to a couple of ancient texts," she says, referring to the Yoga Sutras. "This is just a tiny sliver of what exists in Indian philosophy and even specifically yoga philosophy," she adds. "This is why the discussion of legitimacy in yoga is extremely irrelevant, because we don't know what [the sutras'] role was at the time. How important they were, how many people read them, how they were used and how they compared to other texts or other philosophies that may have been used at the same time."

To someone like Kadetsky, looking to yoga's past to solve the problems of yoga's ever-evolving future makes as much sense as using the Bible to convince people that dinosaurs and man once coexisted. ("Like the Flintstones?" as *The Sopranos'* Tony once pithily queried.) But whether it makes sense or not is almost beside the point. The yamas are the ethical yardstick for yoga. Without them we have no other way of judging how wide the gap between yoga principles and yoga practice has become. So let's really examine the yoga industry by exploring each of the yamas in depth and in context. Cynics might say that's like giving yoga enough rope to hang itself.

7

Chasing a Yoga Butt

*Yoga helps endure what cannot be cured and cure
what need not be endured.*
—B.K.S. IYENGAR, QUOTED IN AMY LABBE, "FROM
ASANA TO PRANAYAMA"

As if it needed saying, the world is a violent and often terrible place. The twentieth century was particularly and spectacularly dreadful, with humans unleashing more organized chaos and killing on one another in greater numbers than all the past centuries combined. Casualties from World War Two alone, the greatest man-made disaster of all time, have been estimated at between 50 and 70 million people. And with war, genocide, torture and imprisonment continuing at an alarming pace, it appears that the twenty-first century may not be very different. Man, it seems, has and always did have an insatiable lust for self-destruction.

The people of ancient India understood this. Of the three major religions that originated in the region, Hinduism, Buddhism and Jainism, all have as a core teaching the notion of ahimsa, the code of conduct that prohibits the killing or injuring of sentient beings. The roots of ahimsa can be found in many ancient religious texts, such as the Vedas, Upanishads, Dharma Shastras and the Mahabharata. And around 200 B.C., Patanjali, in his Yoga Sutras, identified ahimsa as the first yoga yama, the foremost yogic teaching, with all other teachings building on its practice.

Thou Shalt Not Harm

Derived from the Sanskrit root word *himsa,* meaning "violence," *ahimsa* translated literally means "nonviolence," the avoidance of violence. In yogic and Hindu philosophy it has come to have a wider definition, meaning to abstain from harming any sentient being in thought, word or deed in order to release all hostility and to lose the desire to do injury. It can be thought of as a Hindu equivalent of Christianity's Golden Rule. "It's kind of the foundation moral principle of the world's major spiritual traditions," says Lamb. In the past two hundred years, influential Indian religious leaders such as Swami Vivekananda, Ramana Maharishi and, most significantly, Mahatma Gandhi, have espoused the importance of ahimsa. Seen as a paragon of Hindu piety and wisdom, Gandhi lived his life guided by the principle of ahimsa, believing it to be the most powerful force in existence and the highest law of humankind. Ahimsa has been the inspiration for countless movements since Gandhi's day, from Dr. Martin Luther King's nonviolent civil rights protests through to the campaign for vegetarianism and veganism.

In yoga, the practitioner's "treatment of self" is an important aspect of ahimsa, perhaps the most important part. "We should take the approach of not harming *ourselves,*" says Lamb. Watch a typical yoga class, however, and you'll see ahimsa go out the window pretty swiftly. Driven by our Western obsession with physical beauty, strength and agility, many yogis are routinely harming themselves by pushing their bodies to their physical edge. The number of yoga-related injuries has spiked in recent years, especially in North America. According to the U.S. Consumer Product Safety Commission, there were over five thousand yoga-related injuries in 2005, an increase of more than thirteen hundred cases from the previous year. In fact, for the three years up to October 2007, over thirteen thousand Americans were treated in an emergency room or a doctor's office for yoga-related injuries, with the cost of treating these injuries coming to nearly $90 million in 2005 alone, according to the commission. A Florida-based orthopedic surgeon told

Newsweek he sees "three or four cases a week."[1] A Calgary-based yoga teacher and kinesiologist holds popular seminars on how to prevent yoga injuries.[2]

Dr. Robert Gotlin is sports rehab director at Beth Israel Medical Center in New York and host of *Dr. Rob Says,* a health and fitness show on ESPN radio. He says a simple case of "keeping up with the Joneses" is causing many of these injuries: "People oftentimes, in a studio setting, look at the person next to them and ... say, 'Why can't I? I'm going to push harder.' Getting to that point may be okay for the person next to you, but not for you. You've got to keep that in perspective."[3] Gotlin is careful to point out that the number of yoga injuries is relatively small compared with those from recreational sports, yet he admits the number has skyrocketed, particularly knee and back injuries from yoga. "A muscle can become more flexible and improve its elasticity and flexibility, but there is a limit. A muscle can only stretch so far," he says. Going beyond that point "could begin to damage the muscle's inherent structure, which holds it together. Once you damage that inherent structure, you damage the muscle." To Lamb, injuring yourself doing yoga is lunacy. "We have people in our twenties now who are getting degenerative discs from doing too deep backbends, just so they can do a deeper one than they did the day before. That's not yoga. That's something else. Yoga would never ask that of you," she says.

Reports indicate that yoga performed in a heated environment is the most detrimental.[4] It's long been known that Bikram Yoga and other hot styles attract the most competitive and most enthusiastic yogis, the classic type A's. "The weekend warriors," as Gotlin describes them, "see this as their outlet to focus their ninety minutes, their hour of time, to give all they've got. And they will go overboard." The heat and intensity that make up the hot yoga experience contribute to the problems. "Because you feel warm, because you're in an environment where your psyche is so attuned, and because your endorphins are flowing, you don't realize that you're overstretching a muscle. And you cause damage," Gotlin says. As Lamb says, "People have wonderful short-term benefits from it. I know people who have been practicing Bikram Yoga for years who are just the picture of health." But without any real scientific assessment, she's hesitant to believe the benefits are worth the risk. "We don't know the long-term effect of raising the core body temperature daily on a long-term basis," she says. According to Dr. Gotlin, "The message is, just be careful. Be aware and ask questions. Don't be fearful to say, 'I can't do that.'"

The problem here is that hot yoga styles virtually *require* students to continually work at the very edge of their capability. In Bikram Yoga each posture is performed twice, with practitioners commanded to "go deeper" into the pose the second time. I can personally attest that, for beginners, it can be a grueling and even painful experience. Instructors, meanwhile, often brush off discomfort and nausea as something the yogi can work through. "There shouldn't be pain associated with yoga. Yes, you may reach an edge physically, and you have to learn how to work with it, but you shouldn't push yourself," cautions Lamb.

Christine Drabek has been doing Bikram Yoga since 2004, primarily to remedy lower-back problems. Almost twenty years after an accident she'd had in her late teens, she still experienced discomfort that made sitting through a long movie painful. She was soon practicing at least three times a week, a typical trajectory for Bikram yogis. "Once I got into it, I got *really* into it," she tells me.[5] Although Christine occasionally manages to bring her sister Amy along for class, Amy doesn't share her sibling's enthusiasm for Bikram Yoga. "I'm not a fan," she says. "I would never come without Christine." Amy is concerned that her sister may be pushing herself too hard. "You have to know your limits. You have to know that pain is no good," she says. "If something hurts, I'm going to stop doing it. I don't care if means that I'm not going to go 'deeper.'"

Many neophytes, however, don't know when to stop, even when they're light-headed and feeling nauseated. "I know there are some claims made that when you practice in the hot room, if you get nauseated it's because you're purifying and releasing toxins. The more likely story is that that you're becoming dehydrated and it's the early stages of heat exhaustion," says Lamb. Dr. Gotlin agrees. "Dizziness, to me, connotes either dehydration or overexertion," he says. "We can wind up having cardiac issues where we have arrhythmia, or abnormal heart beats. The arrhythmias can be serious." According to Lamb, there has been at least one report of a fatal heart attack during a hot yoga class, although she's quick to point out the victim was overweight and middle-aged and may have had high blood pressure. (Not good on the word-of-mouth front, though.) Gotlin's advice is to just be certain of what you're getting into: "Most of us are apt to being open-minded, to trying something, to doing something without having the foresight to understand that it may not be the right thing. We fall victim to a sales pitch, good advertising, or a good concept and don't understand, really, the details."

Dehydration is more of a concern in Bikram Yoga than in other styles because students are specifically told to *avoid* drinking water until about twenty-five minutes into the class. The reasons are twofold, according to Bikram. First, so the body can warm up from the inside out, and second, because water can be a distraction. The student's energy is on the water and not the postures, so the theory goes. Additionally, drinking water while others are midposture is considered interfering with the energy of the class, so many Bikram yogis risk dehydration rather than disrupt others. "That is part of the practice that I dislike. They sort of in a punitive way tell you what you can or can't do in a class," Christine says. While she still struggles with the heat, she says other practitioners don't bat an eyelash, seeing their refusal to drink water as a badge of honor.

Like many people, Christine found her curiosity had been tweaked by the idea of yoga as physical therapy, an aspect of the practice that has become increasingly significant during the past decade. Words such as *rehabilitative* and *restorative* are now routinely used to advertise yoga. This has even fueled the rise of a new field, yoga therapy, one-on-one yoga classes in which the poses are tailored to target an individual's specific injuries and trouble spots. In May 2007 *The New York Times* claimed that membership in the International Association of Yoga Therapists had in three years tripled from 760 to 2060. (The article was otherwise fairly disparaging, raising concerns that the yoga therapy industry has no formal training or standards. "Buyer beware. I've seen some strange things done in the name of yoga therapy," one yoga therapist was quoted as saying. "I have certainly seen patients asked to do positions that have made them worse," an orthopedic surgeon said.)[6] Interest in yoga-as-therapy is of increasing interest to the medical community. The Albert Einstein College of Medicine in New York has been running a study since 2001 to determine if yoga can help reduce the physical and emotional side effects of living with cancer or its treatment.[7] The Johns Hopkins Arthritis Center has a study probing how yoga may benefit people with arthritis.[8]

All this got me thinking about an entirely unscientific experiment. I wanted to see how an intensive five-week, four-class-a-week Bikram Yoga schedule might affect somebody's mental and physical well-being. Would we see vast improvement? Christine Drabek seemed like the perfect candidate and agreed to take part. Our first step was visiting Dr. Gotlin at Beth Israel for a thorough physical, to establish Christine's physical baseline. Like many other hot yogis he sees, Christine says she's been getting headaches ever since she began Bikram Yoga. "The three or four months when I first started were just overwhelming," Christine recalled. "Usually you have a thing of Advil in your cabinet for a year," she said. "I was going through bottles of it." She also explained that certain postures were causing her pain. Gotlin's advice about the headaches, the same advice he gives all hot yogis, was to avoid dehydration by drinking plenty of water whenever Christine felt she needed it—despite what her Bikram instructor might say. And he warned her to be careful to not overstretch in any position where she felt discomfort—again despite what her instructor might say.

Of course, Christine didn't just get into Bikram Yoga to remedy her lower-back pain. "I wanted to lose some weight," she says. She was egged on by the example of her mother and sister: "They are both very slim and they've lost a lot of weight through yoga. I've struggled with my weight."

Om Improvement

It's the one pitch that has more people coming through the door than any other, the idea that you can transform your body through yoga. The tyranny that physical beauty exerts over society is perhaps more at work in the yoga studio than anywhere else. "Yoga has

The Dharma Diet

It may not be what the yogis of old had in mind, but shedding extra pounds is one of the main reasons modern yogis come to class. But is yoga really the fast track to weight loss that it's cracked up to be? Don't be fooled by all those rail-thin yogis; the question is more complicated than it seems. Weight loss and gain are complicated processes, affected by all sorts of disparate factors, such as lifestyle, willpower and genetics. While it's true that yoga helps to lengthen, strengthen and tone muscle, muscle weighs more than fat, thus sculpting the body is not the same as losing weight (no matter how good "the new you" looks naked). Also keep in mind the style of yoga being practiced. Slow, contemplative yoga styles offer little in the way of an aerobic workout. The extremely physical and "hot" yoga styles, meanwhile, burn more calories but often at a hidden cost, according to Beth Israel's Dr. Robert Gotlin. Rather than losing body fat—the key to real weight loss—power yogis may merely be shedding water weight. "And that's not what we're looking for. We want to maintain the water because the body needs water," Gotlin says. "People who are losing the weight might be leaning toward dehydration."

Some of the facts about yoga and weight loss may be dispiriting, but that hasn't stopped plenty of books on the subject from flooding the market. Just browsing through some of these wordy titles can be a workout in itself. There's *Fat Free Yoga— Lose Weight & Feel Great FOR BEGINNERS & BEYOND*, *Yoga for Weight-loss: The Effective 4-week Slimming Plan for Body, Mind and Spirit*, *Yoga Fights Flab: A 30-Day Program to Tone, Trim and Flatten Your Trouble Spots*, and *Yoga Turns Back the Clock: The Unique Total-Body Program That Fights Fat, Wrinkles and Fatigue*.

become about beautification of the body and health of the body in the West, when there is so much more to it," says Trisha Lamb, an irony she likens to "stepping over vast treasure to pick up pennies."

And as weight loss continues to trump spiritual gain, a peculiar and even grotesque downside has emerged.

In 2005 *The Guardian* newspaper in England reported on a disturbing increase in eating disorders among adherents of high-energy yoga workouts, particularly Ashtanga style. "That is the appeal of ashtanga, because it feels like real exercise. You sweat and you feel the exertion," the article quoted one twenty-five-year-old man saying. "It works as a safety net," he added. "If I do have a lapse [overeat], I have this practice to get rid of those extra calories." A young woman drew parallels between the emotions generated by both yoga and anorexia. "Not eating is like an addiction, because you feel nothing is going to harm you," the young woman said. "You feel clear and blissful and completely unattached—which, of course, is also what I was trying to achieve through yoga." Another young woman with an eating disorder had the sense to know that yoga pushed the wrong buttons for her. "Because I'd been anorexic and had had lots of problems with addiction, it was really unhealthy for me," she said.[9]

Yoga protocol can also spark some of the compulsive behaviors associated with eating disorders. For instance, most yoga styles ask that you practice on an empty stomach. This is great cover for someone with anorexic tendencies who's already trying to avoid food. Yogis also have a penchant for strictly controlling their diet. Competitive yogi Esak Garcia adopted a strict raw-food diet for two months prior to competing in a yoga championship. "That definitely changed my practice a lot. I got much more flexible after that," he says. "But I had to stop doing raw foods because I was losing too much weight. I was getting emaciated." (Interestingly, the food obsession shared by so many Bikram yogis is not shared by Bikram himself, who eschews what he calls "goat food" for "people food"—steak, pizza, french fries and Coke.)

Competition among yogis can also enable compulsive behaviors. Because being thin is often equated with being flexible, and because everybody wants a deeper stretch, the pressure is on to keep the body lean and mean. An absurd notion has also evolved that being flexible equates to being spiritual. Nobody wants to lose that race, especially not the type of addictive personality that's often attracted to Power-yoga styles. "We don't want the aerobic aspect of yoga to become another addiction," New York–based yoga instructor Matthew Godino said in a 2007 Columbia Journalism School web article. "The kind of yoga that would work best [for not triggering or enabling an eating disorder] would be a gentler style, something focused on breath work, relaxation and meditation."[10]

The trend toward anorexia and distorted body images is more disturbing given that yoga has been seen in the past as a way to *overcome* such disorders. There's a reason yoga has become a staple at eating-disorder clinics across North America. Through yoga, people can connect with their bodies and focus on what the body is capable of, hopefully in turn de-emphasizing concerns about what the body looks like. Godino can attest to this process. He was a classic anorexic, weighing at one point just eighty-eight pounds, before using yoga to recover. "Yoga has given me the tools to meet life's challenges more effectively," he said. "So instead of turning to food or to an addictive process like starving, I have a healthy alternative." Chef and teacher Mary Taylor also used yoga to overcome an eating disorder, turning that insight into a book, cowritten with Lynn Ginsburg, titled *What Are You Hungry For? Women, Food, and Spirituality.* Taylor believes body image and eating disorders are often symptoms of a spiritual void, and she uses yoga and meditation to help others overcome their deep-seated food issues.[11]

The dialogue about eating disorders on yoga discussion boards can be illuminating. "Since I have started practicing yoga I do notice that I 'want' to eat. The mental part of anorexia is the most important part to try and overcome, not the weight part," says one member. "There is *nothing* which *yoga* cannot help," says another. Perhaps a member named Christine says it best. "Yoga won't 'cure' anything," she says. "It's up to us and how we use yoga. It remains a tool."[12] This is a point worth emphasizing, and one not expressed often enough in modern yoga circles. Yoga itself is not a treatment. Yoga is merely a technique. It can harm as well as heal. The Greeks said it best: All things in moderation.

So what happened to Christine's body after five weeks of intensive yoga practice? During a visit to Dr. Gotlin's office, she reported feeling more energetic and more focused. She explained that as a result of his advice to stay hydrated, her headaches were almost gone. And she had been careful not to overdo it in any of the painful postures, despite the repercussions. "There was one teacher who said, 'You're not doing the posture.' But for me, I'm doing the posture," she explained. Dr. Gotlin was pleased. "The key for it being good for you is that you're guiding the exercise, you're not being guided by someone else. You're being instructed, but you know your limitations. That's the key," he said.

All seemed well. But one thing still nagged Christine. "I haven't dropped as much weight as some of the other people I've been practicing with," she said. "I'm a little surprised I haven't made a bit more progress." Here was a woman who had transformed herself in so many ways, yet she remained obsessed with her weight. "I've always had a quick metabolism. I wonder if it slowed my metabolism down, because I haven't lost any weight," she said to me. And later, "I also wonder about water weight. I wonder if I'm retaining water with the amount that I'm drinking."

All things in moderation.

Many yogis, it seems, don't know enough about ahimsa to stop pushing their bodies beyond the limit. Not a problem. That's why we have yoga instructors. The yoga instructor is a highly skilled professional, trained to understand how the human body works, how each individual body is unique. It's the instructor's job to provide a safe environment in which the yoga students can further their practice. They know when to push, *why* to push, and when enough is enough. That's the idea, anyway. The reality is different. Many yoga teachers are poorly trained and ill-equipped to deal with the wide range of issues that the typical yoga class throws up.

Traditionally, yoga was taught one to one, from guru to disciple, over a number of years. The transmission of yogic knowledge is no longer a time-consuming burden. It's become a reliable and often very profitable side business. Almost all brand-name yoga studios now offer some sort of training program. And who can blame them? It's a seller's market. The need for yoga teachers has exploded over the last decade as yoga's popularity has soared. Teacher training also makes good business sense. In an increasingly cutthroat and volatile environment, the income from yoga classes alone is not enough for most studios to survive on. Training teachers offers an additional, stable income stream. "Here are these people opening their yoga studios," says Anne Libby, former manager of a New York City hot yoga studio. "After a while they're like, 'Jeez, I can't support my business out of the open classes I've got. I know, for $3000 I can train a new teacher!' Fifty of those times three thousand, that's $150,000."[13]

Once she was certain she'd be opening her own studio, Cyndi Lee, owner of Om Yoga in New York, began training ten teachers. "When I opened the studio, I had ten people that were already trained in this style. So it was great. Then more people asked me. They wanted to do teacher training and it just grew from there," she says. Om now offers different levels of training, from five-hundred-hour comprehensive training to sixty-hour refresher courses. "We have the Warrior Weekend, where they come on weekends. We have Joining Heaven and Earth, where they come twice a week for four months," she says.

But the demand for teachers has also caused problems, especially in North America. Without a governing body to oversee the process, the standards vary widely from training to training. Certification programs range in length from two years to just two days—with the "quickie" training increasing in popularity all the time. "You have a number of people in this country who have gotten a yoga teacher's certification in a weekend. There's no way that you can cover the depth of yoga philosophy in a weekend," says Trisha Lamb. "Yoga is such a vast discipline," says Tony Sanchez, director of Mexico's Academia de Yoga. "You require a little more than two weeks to really comprehend how yoga originated, how it has developed, and how yoga has evolved into what it is now."

The Yoga Alliance, perhaps the closest thing American yoga has to a governing body, has set a minimum standard of two hundred hours of training for basic certification and five hundred hours for advanced certification. Yoga groups in the United States and Canada generally stick to these guidelines. Yet there's no obligation or requirement for training programs to run this allotted time. In fact, there's no requirement that yoga teachers be trained at all. "Anyone can call him- or herself a yoga teacher without any training whatso-ever," says Lamb. And that's just what's happening. According to *Time* magazine, only about sixteen thousand of the estimated sev-enty thousand instructors in the United States are even certified.[14]

It's not only *how* but *what* wannabe yoga teachers are being taught that's come under scrutiny. Comprehensive teacher training should cover yoga philosophy, ethics and history, not just postures and meditation. In quickie courses, you're lucky to get beyond lotus pose. "There are too many people out there throwing together teacher-training programs and training teachers. I really think there should be higher standards," says Marilyn Barnett, who ran a studio with Anne Libby in downtown New York. "[The teachers] are learning some key things that they're throwing around, but they really haven't embodied it," she says.[15] Tony Sanchez agrees. "I think a lot of people are going into the discipline without really having enough instruction, without having enough discipline, and without paying their dues," he says. "They don't really have the knowledge that gets acquired only through discipline."

Rodney Yee describes the teacher-training world as a pyramid. At the top are highly trained, well-respected teachers with more than thirty years' experience. The middle of the pyramid, where most teachers reside, is made up of well-trained and certainly competent professionals. But the teacher who received his or her training in a weekend or at a two-week retreat? "The bottom dweller of the pyramid," Yee says. "I don't care how much of a genius you are and how much you study in one month. There's not enough time to absorb information.... The body doesn't work that way. The brain doesn't work that way."

Let's be clear that the would-be teachers aren't to blame for poor training. Many of them see teaching yoga as a calling and are eager to begin. If someone can offer them a certificate after just two days that can help them land a job, why not take it? After all, unless they have a following or name recognition, teaching yoga is hardly a road paved with gold. Few studios offer their teachers benefits. There's little long-term job security. And it can take a long time to carve out a niche. "If you average $50 a class, you're not making survival rate wages here in New York City," says Anne Libby. She adds that with the inevitable glut of new teachers, everyone is looking within the same small number of jobs. "It creates a situation of desperation," she says. "If you're thinking that you're going to become rich and famous and a big deal from teaching yoga," says Cyndi Lee, "you're going to be disappointed." And financially struggling teachers often feel compelled to jam their classes with as many paying customers as possible. "Yoga is supposed to be about a relationship you have between teacher and student. If you have fifty students in a class and you're teaching eight classes," Libby claims, "that's not a relationship. That's promiscuity."

Which all gets back to my main point: how all of this affects ahimsa, the edict of non-harming. The answer is, not well. For instance, teachers without proper training are the ones most likely to breach little-understood ethical guidelines. In a web article titled "Yoga's Silent Scandal," *Whole Life Times* reported on the rising number of yoga instructors sleeping with their students. The article quoted Judith Lasater, president of the California Yoga Teachers Association and a leader in the push for ethics in yoga, on the edict of ahimsa. "It's very much akin to the medical 'First do no harm' directive," she said. "It's almost impossible as a teacher to become intimately involved with a student and not create suffering." The article also quoted yoga-studio owner and author Janice Gates, who heard repeated accounts of teacher-student affairs during interviews she conducted for her book *Yogini,* a collection of stories exploring the role of women in yoga. "A male teacher in a room full of mostly women, dressed in tight clothing, moving, breathing and sweating—all looking to him for direction. Most teacher-training programs simply don't prepare them to handle that skillfully," Gates said.[16] Poorly trained teachers are also more likely to bring their personal baggage into class. And that, according to Anne Libby, can adversely affect their primary reason for being there in the first place. "These are people who are supposed to be offering a spiritual lesson," she says. "How many of them have received the level of training that allows them to *not* bring their survival needs into the classroom?" she wonders.

Most troubling, however, is the potential for a poorly trained teacher to cause or allow a student to be physically harmed simply because the student is trying to do a better backbend than yesterday. "If you're really creasing your back when you do a backbend, you're damaging yourself. You have to have teachers who are well trained," says Lamb. "Without well-trained teachers, you can almost guarantee that you're going to have accidents, problems, permanent injuries, etcetera," she says.

"In a yoga practice you do more body engineering than a typical chiropractor will do over the course of a year. So to put that into the hands of an untrained person who has had only a few weekends of trainings and has all sorts of creative ideas about anatomy, physiology and people's conditions, that's a fairly risky endeavor," says Rob Wrubel, cofounder of Yoga Works. Yoga Works instructors complete rigorous training before being coupled with a senior instructor for mentoring, Wrubel says. "When someone with scoliosis who is sixty years old shows up in your class and you're doing inversions, you'd better know exactly what modifications of the poses you can do. A lot of the time that doesn't happen."

Even the most well-trained teachers may not always do their best by students. There's been a long-running debate in yoga circles over whether to lock the knee in standing poses. In Bikram Yoga, for example, standing-head-to-knee pose is done with a locked knee ("solid, one piece, concrete, like a lamppost," as Bikram's class dialogue dictates). However, Tony Sanchez, who was taught by Bikram and ran his own hot yoga studio in San Francisco for over twenty years, tells students to keep a slight bend in the knee, to prevent hyperextension. "Gradually, you build up the strength on the tendons, ligaments, and muscles to be able to come up with the proper alignment. Hyperextension will damage the knee in a very gradual but progressive way," Sanchez says. Dr. Gotlin at the Beth Israel Sports Rehab Center shares his opinion. "By flexing that knee way back as hard as you can, you're really jamming that bone," he says. "It's not good for you." But Sanchez had little luck getting Bikram to change his ways, even after presenting him with evidence that a locked knee could cause cartilage damage. "And he did agree with it. And he tried to make these changes. But then all the people that he had trained to hyperextend and lock the knees got totally upset and frustrated. So they ganged up on Bikram and made him go back to his old ways!" Sanchez says with a laugh. To this day Bikram's standing-head-to-knee pose is performed with a locked knee.

It seems clear that ahimsa is not being well practiced within the yoga studio. But what about in the wider yoga world? What harm are yogis are causing each *other*? Capitalism is the story of winners and losers. In a highly competitive environment such as the yoga industry, it goes without saying that studios may have to inflict some "harm" on others to succeed. In this yoga version of prosperity gospel, the new mantra is "Be successful"—even if you have to trample other yogis to succeed. "If we are devoting ourselves to a life of service, then we [yogis] … should have an open mind to be able to see what the next guy is doing," says Tony Sanchez. "Instead of always saying, 'My yoga is the best. Everybody else's yoga is terrible.'"

So just how downward-dog eat downward-dog are we willing to be to succeed? *Yoga Journal,* the largest-circulation yoga magazine in the United States, has been singled out in the past for allegedly unyogic behavior. In a 2002 *Business 2.0* article, writer Paul Keegan described *Yoga Journal*'s behavior in trying to gain a monopoly over the yoga conference circuit as thuggish. The article detailed yoga teacher Jonny Kest's plan to hold a yoga and wellness conference in Michigan, "only to discover how little ahimsa was being practiced back at *Yoga Journal.*" Kest claimed *Yoga Journal* tried to essentially run him out of town by holding a similar conference just fifty miles away within weeks of his event.[17]

John Abbott, *Yoga Journal* publisher and CEO at the time, interprets events differently: "[Keegan] was insinuating that there were predatory or unfair practices, and he didn't really point any out. There was no validity to the insinuation. To think that big portions of the United States will be staked out and owned by someone because they happen to have a yoga event there, which was the implication in the article, is certainly not consistent with reasonable business practices in the United States."

Yoga Journal has been a surprise success under Abbott's watch. A former investment banker at Citicorp and an avid yoga practitioner, he bought the magazine in November 1998, when circulation was under 90,000. He soon took over as CEO and publisher, installing a new editor-in-chief. In January 2000 Abbott's team redesigned and relaunched the magazine. Paid circulation has since grown to 350,000, with a readership of over a million people. (In September 2006 the magazine was bought by Active Interest Media, which publishes *Vegetarian Times, Southwest Art* and other "consumer enthusiast" titles.) "*Yoga Journal* existed for many years right on the edge of near bankruptcy," Abbott says, adding that it may never be a spectacular financial juggernaut. "Are we going to make lots of money? No, we're not going to, this isn't the type of thing where you make lots and lots of money. But we should make a good 10 to 15 percent return."

Abbott's takeover was, by his own admission, quite dramatic, with many long-time staffers openly expressing their fears that the magazine would turn faceless and corporate. "The former owners came and had a big staff meeting and announced to the staff that they had enticed me to come be the new publisher and owner. And there were catcalls and yelling, and a couple of women left crying. This was disastrous from their perspective," he says. Today only one employee from before Abbott's arrival remains on staff. It's possible that Abbott is in the critics' headlights because of the magazine's success. Or, as Abbott concedes, running a business may not always be compatible with ahimsa in its purest form. "In our highly commercial U.S. free-enterprise system there's going to be stuff that transgresses what you would like. But I see it as part of our mission … to toe the line," he says. He also believes there's a "heightened sensitivity" to working in the yoga world. "You often receive a righteous outcry, a moralistic interpretation of what we're doing. We listen and decide what we should do. And the litmus test is, does it really live up to this integrity bar?"

Yoga Wars

Talk to Marilyn Barnett about integrity and ahimsa. In 1997, in a compact two-level space just blocks from the World Trade Center, Barnett opened Yoga Connection NYC, the first hot yoga studio in New York City. (Although she trained with Bikram Choudhury, Barnett chose to open a studio outside the Bikram franchise.) This hot new workout was an immediate success. "It was attracting not just people who like yoga but people that wouldn't even *consider* yoga. And it was kind of different. We grew really rapidly," Barnett says. By 2000 another Bikram studio had opened—the first of what would be a bumper crop. "Another one opened, like, within nine months after that or a year after that. Then it just started really going crazy," Barnett recalls. "That was still good, because it was still getting the word out there to more and more people. *Everybody* was really busy. In fact, we had to cut our classes off because it was too full." By 2003 the situation in New York had gotten insane. According to Barnett's partner, Anne Libby, "a yoga studio opened in Manhattan about every six to eight weeks." Inside this insular environment the atmosphere was getting tense, says Barnett. "They were opening a little too close for comfort. It was sad, because I know all these people. They were my students before they were teachers."

September 11 delivered an even bigger shock for the tiny studio in the shadow of the Twin Towers. At first the studio filled a small and immediate need. Libby remembers "having people come off the trade center site to come in and take class. I remember one guy who was an engineer who worked all night on a site and came to our 6:45 A.M. class. He came in and his clothes and he were covered with dust. We were like, 'Come on in and take class.' " When the dust did settle, however, things were different. "Everyone was freaked out. Nobody knew what was happening. We didn't know which students were not coming back because they *couldn't* come back," Libby says. In that decimated, depressed environment, the studio struggled. "We lost our whole foundation," Barnett says. The partners fought back, working hard to attract yogis from outside the neighborhood and offering support, deals and incentives to those who remained. Eventually, the business was operational again.

The final nail in Yoga Connection's coffin came when a new Equinox gym in the neighborhood started offering yoga. "When the big gym down the street from us opened," Barnett says, "our income went to half, like that," snapping her fingers for effect. She shakes her head at the situation she'd found herself in. "Without having the numbers of people and the classes be full, it's very hard to make ends meet."

The studio was now behind in its rent and summer was approaching, traditionally a slow period. So, like many New Yorkers in a real-estate bind, Barnett went to her last resort; she made an appeal to her landlord, telling him she was having a hard time getting back on her feet and warning him he might want to consider looking for a new tenant. She thought the process might take a few months. But this is New York. A prospective new tenant was already waiting. This tenant knew all about the space. This tenant liked that it was a yoga studio. And this tenant was ready to move, now. Suddenly, Barnett had a month to clear out. And the mysterious tenant who just happened to be waiting in the wings, ready to jump at the chance to take over Barnett's space? "It was someone who taught for me," she says. Ouch.

It's the last day of business at Yoga Connection. "I actually feel calm. I feel calm and sad, but somewhat relieved," Barnett says. She has one last class to teach, and the place is packed. The irony is not lost on her. "I haven't been in a room this full in a while!" she says with a laugh. "Is there room for me?" The class is routine, as always. People bend, stretch and sweat. But an air of sadness, of finality, hangs over the room. Ninety minutes later it's all over. "Thank you for allowing me to teach," Barnett says simply, before leaving the room, tears welling in her eyes. In the lobby, students take their last chance to thank her, to say goodbye and to offer compliments and condolences. Barnett is philosophical. "It is what it is. There's just a time, sometimes, that things come to an end. It doesn't mean our yoga came to an end," she says. And she's positive about the new studio going up in her space. "I think it's great that there will be a hot yoga studio down here for the people who want to continue doing it." She doubts, however, that there will be any relationship between her and her former teacher/new studio owner. "It wasn't like we were friends that hung out together or anything. She was one of my teachers. She's a nice girl and a good teacher," Barnett says. "I mean, good luck. I did everything I could to make the business go. It's like … good luck."

Anne Libby, meanwhile, can't see the sense in opening another yoga studio in the same space. "Lower Manhattan below Canal

Street has thirty thousand residents. If you get 1 percent of that market, that's three hundred people. Three hundred people, in my opinion, can barely support a yoga studio. Now they're splitting it across every gym and five yoga studios. How could that make sense? Would you, as an investor, look at that situation and say, 'Okay, I think I'll open another yoga studio in that space?'"

"I know that some of the smaller studios are closing their doors," says Cyndi Lee, owner of Om Yoga. "I also know quite a few studios that have popped up in the last couple of months. So, there are opportunities," she adds. One wonders just how long Lee can hold that hopeful note. Om exists in a neighborhood awash in yoga studios. Just one block away is the Jivamukti headquarters. In that same building is a Bikram Yoga studio. Yogi Bhajan's Kundalini Yoga organization has an East Coast headquarters just three more blocks away. Yoga Works is fewer than seven blocks away. Om Yoga could just as easily be swallowed up and spit out, just like Yoga Connection or any number of other players have been.

"We are so divided," laments Tony Sanchez, director of Mexico's Academia de Yoga. "Yoga is supposed to be reuniting people. It should not be making us more competitive and more aggressive, more greedy, you know?"

Forget ahimsa. Isn't this sort of thing just plain *uncool*? Anne Libby refuses to take that bait. For her the important thing is that yoga itself survives. "It's not really about us, is it?" she says. "Our students will find other places to practice yoga. Those teachings will survive anything that happens in business. Five thousand years of survival, that's truth." It's a good point. Should we have more sympathy for Barnett and Libby than for any other small-business owner struggling in New York, simply because they're yogis? Opportunism and competitiveness are the engines that drive Western capitalism, after all. Yet there is a sad irony to the Yoga Connection case, a small illustration of an industry that seems to have forgotten its golden rule. Barnett's well-regarded little yoga studio survived fickle, fussy New Yorkers, constant rent hikes and even a terrorist attack. What it could *not* survive were other yogis.

A final note for you neo-con hawks lurking among all the yoga doves and wondering where you fit in. Fear not. It seems the timidity of ahimsa is not ironclad. In fact, yoga has a whopping vindictive streak, at least according to Dr. David Frawley, director of the American Institute of Vedic Studies, based in New Mexico. In an illuminating and provocative essay titled "Yoga, Ahimsa and the Terrorist Attacks," written shortly after 9/11, Frawley contends that a deeper reading of the yoga tradition reveals a loophole that allows yogis to inflict *some* harm to avoid *greater* harm, "like a surgeon removing a harmful tumour so that it does not grow and damage the whole body." Frawley cites two kinds of ahimsa in the yoga tradition: as a *spiritual* principle, in which nonviolence on all levels is the aim, and as a *political* principle. This latter version of ahimsa allows the use of violence to counter evil forces. This ahimsa is not about appeasing, tolerating or excusing bad or evil behavior. Instead it requires action to reduce harm. Frawley cautions, though, that it "must be done in the right way. The application of force, done wrongly, can make the situation worse." Frawley notes that the acclaimed Indian nationalist and strict yogi Sri Aurobindo supported military action in both World War Two and the Korean War, that in 1998 the Dalai Lama approved of India's nuclear tests and that Gandhi himself in 1947 approved of bringing in the Indian army to deal with plundering bands of terrorists in Kashmir.[18]

This concept may sound familiar. It's something we've heard much about in recent years. Some people call it "just war." Others call it "preemptive war."

8

Stretching the Satya

My uniform experience has convinced me that there
is no other God than Truth.
—MOHANDAS K. GANDHI, *ALL MEN ARE BROTHERS*

In January 2008 the world marked the sixtieth anniversary of
Mahatma Gandhi's death, assassinated by a Hindu extremist. To
many westerners, the life of the man considered India's spiritual and
political conscience offers the most relevant example of the two most
integral yoga yamas, ahimsa and satya, in action. Like most Hindus,
Gandhi believed the two principles went hand in hand. "Ahimsa and
Truth are so intertwined that it is practically impossible to disen-
tangle and separate them," he observed. "Ahimsa is the means; truth
is the end."[1]

Note here that Gandhi uses the basic English translation of *satya,*
"truth." Yet it's important to get the definition exactly right. Like
many Sanskrit words, *satya* carries many meanings and understand-
ings. And as we'll see, a lazy translation can be easily, perhaps pur-
posefully, misunderstood. The word *satya* comes from the root *sat,*
which means "truth." But not truth as in fact, certainty or even hon-
esty. For the religious peoples of ancient India among whom the
term originated, truth meant the ageless, eternal and unchanging
truth of existence, a metaphysical truth with the implication of a

higher order. Adding the Sanskrit suffix *ya* activates the word, resulting in the more commonly accepted meaning of "truthfulness in word and thought."

The twin principles of ahimsa and satya came to define Gandhi's life. Although "passive resistance" had become the popular label for his nonviolent campaigns, most notably for India's independence from Great Britain, Gandhi thought an Indian term would be more appropriate. The result was *satyagraha,* the combination of *satya* with another Sanskrit term, *agraha,* meaning "firmness" or "force." "I thus began to call the Indian movement satyagraha, that is to say, the Force which is born of Truth and Love or nonviolence, and gave up the use of the phrase 'passive resistance,'" Gandhi explained.[2] Gandhi's satyagraha campaigns are almost universally revered, from the first satyagraha in South Africa in 1906 to oppose the country's racist policies to the large-scale satyagraha campaign against the British salt tax in colonial India in 1930. Of course, most resonant was the three-decade-long satyagraha campaign to free a nation of 500 million people from colonial rule. And when Britain, after two hundred years of colonialism, finally granted India independence in 1947, little blood had been spilled. "Every problem would lend itself to solution if we are determined to make the law of truth and non-violence the law of life," Gandhi declared.[3] Gandhi's philosophy of satyagraha soon became a beacon to peaceniks everywhere, forming the backbone of countless crusades against injustice, including Dr. Martin Luther King's nonviolent civil rights movement in the United States.

But the sixtieth anniversary of Gandhi's assassination has also brought about a worldwide reassessment of his effectiveness. Obviously, India's independence was not the work of one man. Millions of Indians yearned for and worked toward change. And some critics, albeit a small minority, have expressed the belief that Gandhi's satyagraha campaigns were in fact ineffectual, perhaps even destructive. Gandhi's peer, the esteemed Indian spiritual leader Sri Aurobindo, who carried the torch of Indian independence at least a decade before Gandhi and who later developed the spiritual path called Integral yoga, was one such critic. "I said that this movement would lead either to a fiasco or to great confusion. And I see no reason to change my opinion," Aurobindo said in 1926. "Only I would like to add that it has led to both."[4]

Even Gandhi's own grandson has raised doubts about his grandfather's legacy. Rajmohan Gandhi has written two biographies of Gandhi: *Gandhi: The Man, His People, and the Empire,* published in 2006, and *The Good Boatman: A Portrait of Gandhi,* published in 1995. Both books have been candid, unflinching examinations of the man and the myth. "The modern Indian or Westerner is not entirely sure that Gandhi's life continues to be a beacon," Gandhi Jr. wrote in a *Washington Post* column in October 1995, around the time *The Good Boatman* was published. "To many, Gandhi might even symbolize ineffective and impractical idealism.... We sense that there was something special about him that might help us in these times, but we are not quite sure what it was, or whether we even want it for ourselves."[5]

If doubts exist about the effectiveness of the world's most prominent practitioner of satya, what are the rest of us to do? One thing is clear: The yoga business is sure struggling with just how far to take this whole truthfulness thing.

Thou Shalt Not Lie

Gandhi, Sri Aurobindo and even Patanjali, the second-century B.C. sage who enshrined satya as the second yama, would likely marvel at how much time today's yoga purists spend defining, looking for and analyzing satya. But ours is a very different satya from the one any of those men might have been familiar with and deserves careful examination. In our postmodern, relativistic culture, the "truth" is often intangible. The truth that Buddhist practitioner Trisha Lamb seeks through yoga is the time-honored and rigorous Sanskrit definition of the word, the truth beyond all knowing, the truth inside us. "We all have a true nature. We're all at some place interested in discovering that," she says. Yoga teacher Diane Featherstone is also working to discover "the self, the deepest truth I have."[6] But Featherstone, who runs a teacher-training program in rural Massachusetts and teaches yoga to corporate America, has no rigid, orthodox interpretation of truth, relying instead on what she calls her "truth filter." "I'm not fixed in my perspective," she says.

Competitive yogi Esak Garcia is also on a quest for truth. "At a young age I really wanted to be rich and make a lot of money and so I set my sights on the Ivy League. But once I got there I was no longer as interested in money. I was more interested in some underlying truth," he says. His search eventually led him to Bikram Yoga.

Also keep in mind that like any good rule, satya is made to be broken. Satya is ideally subservient to ahimsa, the foremost yogic teaching. Thus, it may not always be desirable (let alone smart) to speak the truth, lest our words harm somebody and violate ahimsa. The Mahabharata puts it succinctly: "Speak the truth which is pleasant. Do not speak unpleasant truths." Of course, the Mahabharata also says, "Do not lie, even if the lies are pleasing to the ear. That is the eternal law." No wonder the yoga industry is having such a difficult time.

The spin, hype and hyperbole that fuel capitalism are essential elements for success in today's aggressive yoga industry. Yet it can easily be argued that all of these tactics flagrantly violate the edict of "truthfulness in word and thought." Take the depiction of yoga in popular culture. Yoga magazine covers routinely feature airbrushed photographs of beautiful young women contorted into all sorts of wild and seductive shapes, the kind of shapes (and girls) that are wildly out of reach of the vast majority of yogis. Where are the balding and the paunchy, the middle-aged and out of shape? Arguably those yogis offer a more accurate representation of the modern yoga community. Wouldn't putting *them* on the cover be more in line with satya? "I often have people say, 'Why don't you just have ordinary bodies on the cover?' Well, ordinary bodies just won't sell on the cover. So there's a needle that we thread here," says *Yoga Journal* publisher John Abbott.

Sales or satya? Indeed a difficult choice. And *Yoga Journal* is by no means the only magazine making that choice, merely the most high profile. The fact is, just about every mass-market yoga magazine follows the cute-yogini-as-cover-girl model. Some go one better than yoga hotties and kick it up to yoga celebrities. When *Vanity Fair* ran a photo spread titled "Planet Yoga" in the June 2007 issue, it wasn't Regular Joe Yoga the photographers were following. It was Christy

Turlington, Sting and Rodney Yee. The idea that typical yogis look anything like these perfected specimens is really stretching the satya.

Abbott and his ilk aren't the villains here. It's the yoga consumer who's really to blame. Forget spirituality, say goodbye to satya. It's not yogic philosophy that drives most yogis, it's the pursuit of bodily perfection—the perfect abs, the perfect butt, the perfect backbend. *Yoga Journal,* Abbott says, merely caters to "what our audience tells us they're most interested in. Most people come to yoga through a physical practice. It's quite rare that you find the average people coming to yoga through some pursuit of spirituality." In other words, nobody wants to see ugly people searching for Truth on the cover.

Deciding what came first, the desire for perfection or the depiction of perfection as something to desire, is a classic chicken-and-egg argument. What *is* clear is that yoga and beautiful bodies are now hopelessly intertwined. The message seems to be that yoga is a method that women, mostly, can use to attain physical flawlessness. An article on *elements living* magazine's website about yoga declares the focus is "mind and body harmony" and "a perfect body."[7] *Perfect* body? I don't remember reading that in the Yoga Sutras, but it really does say it all.

It wasn't always thus. A review of past *Yoga Journal* covers unearths a range of interest and imagery. In 1976, a year after the magazine began, "Woodstock guru" Swami Satchidananda graced the cover in all his grizzled glory. In 1985 a playful illustrated cover showed a guru meditating as his own reflection sneered cartoonishly back at him. A 1987 cover showed a young couple holding hands, heads pressed lovingly and earnestly together. A cover from as late as 1995 featured arty shots of opened hands holding rose petals. The covers might have been cheesy, but the ideas they alluded to (The nature of the guru? Interpersonal relationships? The role of flowers?) were at least in keeping with yoga's wide philosophical scope. Those images became a thing of the past in 1998, when John Abbott took over and rebranded the magazine. Now I defy you to find a cover that *doesn't* feature a shapely young woman.

Inside the magazine it's a different story, with a sizable number of articles exploring concerns of the mind and soul. "We are writing about a set of ancient practices that date back several millenniums. These practices have been successful and have lasted because they adapt to the cultural context where they find themselves," Abbott tells me. "In the West yoga is hot.... And I don't think we will be successful in presenting yoga in an accessible fashion unless we package this and make some adaptations to the culture." Abbott gives me a no-nonsense smile. You have to admire him. Although his magazine may not be a paragon of satya, at least his explanation is truthful.

Since its debut in 1982, the bimonthly *Yoga International* has been considered the yoga purists' magazine of choice. The magazine, which bills itself as "the trusted voice of classical yoga," is published and staffed by members of the nonprofit Himalayan Institute ashram in Pennsylvania, founded in 1971 by Swami Rama. (The same Swami Rama found guilty by a jury in 1997 of sexual misconduct after a female adherent claimed he had sexually assaulted her.) "*Yoga Journal* and *Yoga International* are doing different things. We're dedicated to presenting the full range of yoga, and not just yoga in terms of postures or breathing," *Yoga International*'s managing editor, Shannon Sexton, told *Folio* magazine in 2003. "We stress holistic health."[8]

Yoga International has since been redesigned and now publishes under the name *Yoga Plus Joyful Living*. Its circulation has grown, too, from 40,000 in 2000 to over 100,000 readers now, according to the institute's website. The revamped version is slickly packaged and colorfully presented. There are still plenty of articles about "holistic health" ("Meditation Tips That Really Work," "My Retreat to a Mountain Ashram"), although that's not what's most eye-catching. In fact, it's hard to say what I found more enticing, the leggy, lithe beauty doing yoga on the cover or the article about "Perfecting the Lotus Pose."

According to *Folio* magazine's research, *Yoga Plus Joyful Living*'s 76 percent female audience is willing to pay up to 20 percent more for products that "support their lifestyle," such as vitamins, organic foods and yoga apparel.[9] Marketing professionals have a name for this type of consumer: the "inward alternative seeker" or "spiritual spender." Apparently, they must be pretty loose with their wallets, because in recent years the amount of yoga-themed advertising aimed at this group has exploded. It's gone way beyond the products that could claim at least some tenuous link to yoga and healthy living, the low-fat cereals, fitness clubs and the like. Now yoga is used to sell Jeeps, financial services, health insurance plans, Nike shoes and an array of other unrelated products too comically divergent to mention. Again, celebrities have had a hand in fueling this retail orgy. A 2004 TV spot for Gap featuring Madonna, the company's newest spokeswoman, ends with Madge striking a yoga pose in her Gap corduroy pants. The clever campaigns take more liberties: A recent print ad for Hyundai's Sonata sedan featured a woman clad in yoga wear doing a series of yoga poses, the last pose being the "Sonata," in which she assumes the posture of being seated behind the wheel. However, most of these campaigns are inevitably superficial, precisely because the internal, mystical elements of the practice—the search for truth, say—can't be photographed or filmed (although there's surely some smart ad exec trying to figure out how to do that as we speak).

The surge in yoga tops, yoga shoes and all manner of yoga accoutrements even has non-yogis flocking to the registers. "I'm on a community board and one of my colleagues on the board said to me, 'Anne, where can I get yoga pants?'" recalls former New York City yoga studio owner Anne Libby. "She said, 'I don't want to do yoga. But I think the pants are cute.' So there's that element of the business as well." For Libby, some of this merchandise crosses the line. For Trisha Lamb, it's the chakra panties, the minuscule undergarments adorned with one of the body's seven chakras, or energy centers. "The symbol that was on these red bikini panties is sacred to some people," Libby tells me. "I've seen yoga mats that have images of the Buddha on them.... People are putting their feet and their faces and sweating on it. These are the things that are going on," she says, shaking her head in amazement.

Yet the products continue to sell. In this kind of ludicrously receptive retail environment, surely you're an idiot not to be selling *something*. But it's worth remembering here that satya, like all the yamas, works as a *restraint* on behavior. "It is inexpressibly crucial that the yogi make his livelihood only by honest and truthful means," says Swami Nirmalananda Giri, abbot of the traditional Atma Jyoti Hindu monastery in New Mexico. "Selling useless or silly things, convincing people that they need them (or even selling them without convincing them), is a serious breach of truthfulness."[10]

Can an honest yogi honestly defend selling something that no other yogi needs? By that rationale, just about everything on the yoga market would have to go. "You don't need *anything* to do yoga," yoga teacher Diana Featherstone reminds me. "You don't need a $200 pair of Nikes. It'd be nice if you had a mat, but if you don't, bring a towel!" (And I've yet to meet anybody who really *needs* yoga shoes.) "I'm not looking to draw people in with flashy deals. I want them to come because they want to practice yoga," says yoga teacher Marilyn Barnett. The goal, she adds, should never be to "coerce them into buying something that they're not going to use." Of course, it's not that simple—as Barnett and her former business partner Anne Libby learned from experience when their studio in downtown New York folded under financial strain. Meanwhile, they watched other cash-strapped studios survive in part by selling yoga accessories. "If your goal is really to share your teachings," Libby says sadly, "the way things are now, I don't see how you can do it without having some kind of angle that involves selling mats."

Well, there's always sex. If the chakra panties and yoga pants won't get them in the door, the promise of humping like a porn star has been known to move yoga product. Yoga teacher and author Ellen Barrett says the link between yoga and sex has been ignored for too long, and in her new book, *Sexy Yoga: 40 Poses for Mind-Blowing Sex and Greater Intimacy,* she aims to change all that. "Yoga increases flexibility, which helps you to be free and just go for it in sex," Barrett tells *Women's Health* magazine. So *how* does yoga help, exactly? Yoga "breeds confidence," "Makes You Stronger Down Below" and "Gives You Mojo," according to *Women's Health.*[11] And this is just the tip of the, um, iceberg when it comes to the commingling of yoga and sex.

It's hardly news that sex sells. It's no surprise that consumers are more willing to buy something if they think it will make them smell

---

Sex Sells

Sometimes the culture just grabs hold of an idea and runs with it. See if you can spot a theme developing among the following articles found online:

"Yoga and Sex"

"Yoga for Great Sex"

"Yoga for Hotter Sex"

"Yoga Routine for Better Sex"

"Workout: Yoga for Hotter, Better Sex"

"The Big Om—Yoga for a Better Sex Life!"

"4 Yoga Moves for a Better Sex Life"

---

nice or look beautiful or fit or tanned or strong or virile or smart. And it's not a shock to learn advertisers want to open our pockets by enticing us with notions of serenity and contentment, the same reasons many people come to yoga. Manipulating our insecurities, insufficiencies and impoverishments might not reflect the virtuous tradition of satya, but it certainly works. Anyway, all these soft-sell gurus should really be of little concern, considering how many more significant and egregious violations of satya there are to worry about.

The Miracle Workers

An interesting spat broke out recently in Indian yoga circles. In early 2008 popular yoga guru Baba Ramdev got himself in hot water with the Indian Medical Association (IMA) by claiming he'd successfully cured some of his followers of cancer, AIDS and other lethal diseases through the regular practice of pranayama, the control of breath that traditional yogis and attentive readers will recognize as the fourth of Patanjali's eight-limbed path. Ramdev further angered the IMA when, during a subsequent press conference, he allegedly termed doctors "propagators of diseases," claimed they were "encashing on patients' illness" and called for jettisoning conventional medicine in favor of the traditional Indian medical science of ayurveda. National president of the IMA Ashok Adhav responded sharply: "If Baba Ramdev is really sincere, he should visit the cancer hospital here which is flooded with patients and offer his 'magical' treatment free of charge."

A few days later the story took a strange turn. Ramdev held another press conference, this time as part of an "interaction" with IMA members organized by a group of Indian journalists. Ramdev announced he was accepting the IMA's challenge to cure a representative sample of cancer patients. "I have already cured hundreds of patients and presented the medical records of thirty-five of them," he said. Declaring once again that yoga and pranayama can cure some types of cancer, Ramdev said his work would be published in "international medical journals" within three years.[12] I can't wait for that.

She goes by many names. Nirmala Srivastava, Shri Mataji Nirmala Devi, Divine Mother. To many she is simply "Mother," the founder of the religious movement Sahaja yoga, which started in India and now claims centers in almost a hundred countries worldwide. Mother is either saint and sinner, depending on whom you ask. Her followers tout her impeccable personal credentials and point to her high standing in the international community as proof; twice nominated for the Nobel Peace prize; adviser to Gandhi on spiritual matters; from a well-respected, aristocratic family; and married to an Indian diplomat. Some former followers describe her as a cult leader who "claims to grant enlightenment to anyone who asks for it," as one former Sahaja yogi put it. "I am ashamed that I distanced myself from friends and family because I was brainwashed into believing they were negative and that my 'chakras' would 'get caught up' being around non-cult members," the ex-yogi continued.[13] Another ex-Sahaja yogi claims that "devotees worship her, wash her feet and drink the footwash water."[14]

In 1983 Shri Mataji declared she was "Adi Shakti," God in the feminine form. This "simple housewife" turned goddess (a trajectory similar to Australia's Dame Edna Everage, although Edna did it without the miracles) also has the power to heal, it's claimed. In testimonials to the power of Sahaja yoga, followers say Shri Mataji can heal everything from drug addiction to back pain.[15] Others claim to have personally witnessed miraculous cures at the feet of Shri Mataji. On one ardent follower's website, a woman recalls watching Mother cure a sixteen-year-old boy of cancer at Mother's house in London, where she moved in 1974. "I was doing some decorative work, maybe painting or wallpapering, in the same room where Shri Mataji was curing this boy," the woman says. "Shri Mataji gave him healing vibrations on his Nabhi chakra, at the level of his waist.... I saw and felt Shri Mataji cure this boy of cancer. What a tremendous experience."[16] The cures come free of charge and without strings attached—whether you deserve the cure or not, as Shri Mataji seemed to hint at during a 2003 interview with ITV in Ireland. "So many diseases we have cured—cancer, everything. Except for AIDS and this Alzheimer's. Not that we cannot cure, we have cured. But they're extremely rude people, especially these Alzheimer's people are. They abuse you, say all kinds of things. And the other ones think they're martyrs. AIDS people think they're martyrs," she said.[17]

In 1996 Shri Mataji decided to open a hospital. Okay, a "health center," the International Sahaja Yoga Research and Health Centre in Mumbai (formerly Bombay), to be precise. Disease is treated by "vibratory awareness, developed through Sahaja Yoga meditation." The center's website claims that "numerous cases registered have been completely cured. These cases include being cured of infertility, epilepsy, thyroid carcinoma, cancer and many other illness [*sic*]."[18]

It's possible, even likely, that both Shri Mataji and Baba Ramdev are highly empathetic, wildly charismatic, wonderfully idiosyncratic leaders who care deeply about their followers and the rest of humankind. But many yogis, especially those just discovering yoga's philosophical bedrock, have a hard time reconciling the spectacular claims of these gurus or their followers with an ethical precept built on truthfulness. To equate what amounts to stress reduction with a cure for chronic disease sure seems like a whopping misuse of satya, after all. To skeptics these gurus come off looking like the snake-oil salesmen of long-ago country carnivals, peddling homemade potions and new-fangled contraptions. "It's not disingenuous to say that yoga can change your life, because it can. But to claim that it can heal you from cancer, for instance, to make a claim like that is irresponsible," says Trisha Lamb, former head of the California-based Yoga Research and Education Center. "It's certainly a good adjunct therapy. But if someone said, 'You have "X" disease and just doing yoga is going to cure you,' that's an overstatement."

It's often said that the problem here lies with yoga newbies, westerners mostly, who seem to have more at stake in yoga's ancient, spotty wisdoms than actual Indians living a world away. Newbies have the righteous indignation down. It's the skepticism they lack. "The current tendency to idealize India makes it easy to forget the fact that news from the subcontinent of floating yogis or men who could survive for several weeks in airtight boxes used to be greeted with disbelief," yogi and author Elizabeth Kadetsky reminds readers in an interesting online article she wrote titled *Yoga for Skeptics* (perhaps with people like me in mind). "Disbelievers today have set their sights so exclusively on the spectacle of American yoga that they must be reminded that the ground zero of spiritual quackery has always been India," she says.

Of course, you don't need to travel all the way to India to hear fanciful claims about what yoga can do. Indian expatriate Bikram Choudhury has been bragging about the curative effect of his yoga all over North America since he emigrated here over three decades ago. Paul Keegan wrote about the Hollywood hot yoga guru and Kolkata native in 2002 in a fantastically colorful article titled "Yogis Behaving Badly" for the now defunct *Business 2.0* magazine. In the article Bikram compares himself to Jesus Christ and Buddha, says he requires neither food nor sleep and, according to Keegan, "claims to have cured every disease known to humankind." (Further instructive Bikram quotes include "I'm beyond Superman" and—my personal favorite—"I have balls like atom bombs.")[19]

Although Bikram's wild pronouncements might be easy to brush off, the transformations some of his followers have gone through are harder to dismiss. When I first meet Bob Sigmund to discuss his involvement with Bikram Yoga, I offer to help him to his chair. It's amazing that he can walk at all. But Sigmund waves me away, determined to do it alone. He settles into his chair, gives me a smile and jumps right into telling me about "the accident," a horrific car crash Sigmund had when he was just seventeen years old. He was behind the wheel. "I broke the C2 and C6 vertebrae in my neck and I fractured the left central part of my skull and my ear came off. I broke my right clavicle and my left fibula. I was in a coma for six months. I wasn't supposed to walk again," he tells me. "But I was very determined."[20]

Sigmund's attempts at recovery were time-consuming: constant physical therapy, hours on parallel bars and skiing machines. It was frustrating, to say the least. One afternoon a new option presented itself. "I met my friend at a gym and he told me, 'Bob, I'm going to California to learn this yoga and I figure I can help you.' Two months go by. Two years go by. And he never called me. And one day I ran into him. It started from there. He gave me a free year of classes." His recovery since then has been amazing by any reckoning. At a Bikram seminar in New Jersey I watched with astonishment as Sigmund struggled out of his wheelchair to his feet and took long, forceful strides across the stage, before sinking into Bikram's arms. The audience roared their approval. Not every day is that good, Sigmund concedes. "I still fall. I don't even feel it, it just happens. Sometimes I can save myself, but usually I go down like a flash." I remind him that his own doctor never expected he would walk again. Sigmund flashes a broad smile. "Yes."

Mary Jarvis had been teaching Bikram Yoga in San Francisco for ten years when a near-fatal car accident in 1994 left her with herniated disks and cracked vertebrae. Her doctors told her to stay away from rigorous physical exercise such as Bikram Yoga. After six months of dejection, depression and almost constant pain, Jarvis' doctor suggested spinal fusion, grafting the problem vertebrae together to immobilize them, with the hope of reducing or eliminating the pain. But the doctor could not guarantee that she'd be pain-free or that she'd get her flexibility back after the surgery. Jarvis decided to return to yoga instead. After two years of two painful classes a day, she found that the pain began to abate. Fifteen years later she is almost pain-free. Along the way she has become an elder stateswoman of yoga. She now has a flourishing career coaching competitive yogis such as Esak Garcia.

There are so many Bikram recovery stories that the Bikram organization has set up a testimonials page on its website where a litany of loyalists express their heartfelt gratitude to the yoga master for alleviating all manner of ailments. "I owe Bikram for improving my health and for saving my life," says heart-attack victim John. "Bikram gave me my life back and so much more.… He taught me never to give up on myself or any other human being," says Elaine, a hepatitis C sufferer.[21] But Lamb is skeptical that yoga is the magic cure-all people think it is. "The people who practice yoga and see the changes it makes in them become perhaps overly enthusiastic in their proclamations about what it can do," even when their claims "are not well substantiated," she says.

Over the years I've personally heard Bikram declare that his yoga can do everything from helping to restore the use of paralyzed limbs to "curing" hepatitis C. How you *interpret* these assertions depends a lot on definition. "There is no such thing as a cure," an article on Bikram's website states. "When Bikram speaks of curing chronic diseases such as arthritis or slipped disc, he is saying that if you faithfully follow his directions, you will be relieved of your symptoms of discomfort. That is the only 'cure' anyone can offer." However, this cure comes with a few strings attached, or "guarantees," as the website describes them. "Guarantee One: If you continue to perform Bikram's Beginning Yoga Class™ regularly—all twenty-six poses—exactly as directed—the chronic symptoms will not return. Guarantee Two: If you don't continue your Yoga faithfully, fully, or as directed, your symptoms will return."[22] Ouch.

"Can Bikram Yoga actually prevent cancer?" Dr. Joel Brame asks provocatively in an article posted on his website. "Although there are no guarantees, yoga can definitely reduce many of the risk factors of cancer," Brame writes. Brame, who trained as a physician and counselor, says Bikram Yoga helps stave off cancer by reoxygenating the body, bolstering the immune system and "reconnecting the Mind with the Body," among other things.[23] My family history happens to be shot through with cancer. Believe me, I (along with the rest of civilization) would love to find something that prevents this atrocious disease. And I'm more than willing for yoga to be the answer. But the way both Bikram and Brame frame it, we'll never know. Their treatments are infallible because they are impossible to disprove. If I die of something *other* than cancer, is that proof that yoga "prevented" my cancer? Of course not. What if I do happen to die of cancer? Will tests show I didn't do *enough* yoga? People making these kinds of assertions about yoga may mean well, but their claims veer dangerously close to offering false hope, the worst kind of untruth. In the meantime, let's hope they soon find a cure for credulity.

"Yoga is certainly not magic, nor is it the performance of any extraordinary or unusual mystical feat," writes Swami Chidananda, the esteemed spiritual leader and president of the Divine Life Society in India, in a perspicacious essay titled "Yoga: What It Is and What It Is Not." "Behind the deliberate mystification of things pertaining to Yoga there lies a selfish motive," the Swami continues. "Unfortunately, the distortion of this true science is the consequence."[24] Notice his use of the word *science* here. This opens up yet another of the many long-running debates surrounding yoga, a debate of particular importance when we're talking about satya. *Is* yoga a science? Naturally, it depends on whom you ask. In the classical Indian religious texts, yoga is referred to and understood as a science. Swami Chidananda calls yoga "a Religious Science, which means that it goes beyond religion." Notorious (and nuts) seventies guru Bhagwan Shree Rajneesh called yoga "the science of the soul." But none of these definitions encompasses the concept of verifiability that has come to be associated with the word *science*. Dr. Georg Feuerstein, one of the foremost Western authorities on yoga, offers a broader definition that makes more sense. Yoga, he says, "hovers between art and science as well as between science and technology."[25]

The medical community, where excessive prudence is an occupational hazard, has been largely resistant to accepting yoga as science. Yoga-related research occasionally makes an impact on the industry, such as Dr. Dean Ornish's studies in the seventies indicating that yoga combined with diet and meditation can reverse heart disease. Yet despite ample *anecdotal* evidence of what the practice can do, in general yoga research has been seen as peripheral. "Has yoga ever been proven by a scientific study to have cured this or to have helped that?" an American physician who teaches anatomy to aspiring yoga teachers asks me. "The Western physician might say, 'There really isn't enough evidence to recommend that to my patient.'" And a certain percentage of doctors will simply never be won over, she adds. "There is a subgroup of physicians that feel very threatened by anything that is outside the Western medical model." Tony Sanchez, director of Mexico's Academia de Yoga, sees that sort of posturing happening on both sides. He says that in order for yoga to be accepted as a science, it has to work in harmony with other sciences: "If you are using yoga as a science and you are stepping on the other sciences because you believe yoga is superior, you are no longer presenting or offering yoga as a science. You have to be able to incorporate all the elements."

The irony is that while these arguments rage, some of the theories born from yoga are slowly proven true. "There are so many things that ancient yogis used to say about our bodies that just now we're developing the scientific tools to actually measure," the physician tells me. "Science is coming around to validate some of these things." A study published in the *Journal of the American Medical Association,* for instance, found that yoga was more effective than wrist splinting or no treatment in relieving some symptoms of carpal tunnel syndrome.[26] A 2005 study published in the *Annals of Internal Medicine* found yoga is better than traditional exercise in relieving lower-back pain.[27] Studies are proving how effective yoga can be, when combined with the proper diet, in helping people lose weight.

Yet there's just as much that we're finding out through research that simply *isn't* true. Asthma, a common respiratory problem characterized by shortness of breath that is said to affect up to one in four urban children, has always been high on the list of afflictions that yogis of all stripes lay claim to curing. A holistic health website even sells a *Yoga for Asthma* video (fitting neatly into a collection that also includes *Yoga for Menopause, Yoga for Immune Deficiency* and *Yoga for Urinary Tract Disorder*).[28] Even though it's widely believed that the intricate pranayama breathing techniques so integral to yoga can greatly reduce asthma symptoms, recent studies show it to be ineffective at best. A 2003 report published in the medical journal

Thorax stated that a device used to mimic pranayama techniques "does not appear to change bronchial responsiveness or lung function in patients with asthma."[29] A study published in *Thorax* a year earlier looked specifically at the effectiveness of Sahaja yoga in combating asthma. The study concluded that the practice did have limited beneficial effects, mostly in terms of mood and quality-of-life improvements, although little effect on lung function or symptoms was found. The report concluded that further work was required to establish whether Sahaja yoga would be clinically valuable.[30] Not exactly a silver bullet.

In 2007 *Time* magazine reported on the benefits of Facial yoga, stretching exercises for the face that are gaining currency among those who feel plastic surgery is too drastic a step. Accompanying the article was an alarming photo essay depicting some of the poses, including the Satchmo, practiced by puffing your cheeks out, the Marilyn, mastered by blowing kisses, and smiling fish, finessed by pursing your lips. "It's like natural Botox," one workshop leader explained.[31] (This is *Time,* for God's sake!)

Facial yoga is based on the premise that facial muscles will stay toned and thus youthful through exercise. This seems to have about as much theoretical rigor behind it as my mother's admonition to me as a kid not to make funny faces, lest the wind change and I get stuck that way. Mom's advice might have been closer to the truth than even she knew, according to a dermatologist quoted later in the Facial yoga article. "If someone were doing a bizarre contortion, they could spasm. They might actually cause permanent damage," the doctor said. A majority of the experts commenting on Facial yoga in a *New York* magazine article agreed the science was shaky. "Repeated facial expressions and muscle movements cause more wrinkling," one doctor stated. A plastic surgeon cautioned Face yogis to not "strengthen the wrong muscles!" And another plastic surgeon said, "Yoga masters all have svelte, strong bodies, but often narrow, sallow, drooping faces. In short, gravity sucks."[32]

Face it. Facial yoga to combat wrinkles is not all it's cracked up to be. Those of us doing yoga to relieve asthma shouldn't breathe easily just yet. The many people swearing that yoga has cured them should probably wait for verifiable evidence. For yogis to claim miracle cures is simply not in the spirit of satya. More important, yogis need to realize that overstating their cases gets them nowhere. I can attest to the relaxing and rejuvenating qualities of Bikram Yoga and other yoga styles. But has it fixed my dicky knee, rehabbed my troubled coccyx or given me back my zest for life? My rudimentary understanding of satya prevents me from saying anything as definitive as that.

Trial Period

Can yoga cure hot flashes or shell shock? We may never know, but it won't be from a lack of trying to find out. ClinicalTrials.gov is a registry of clinical trials conducted around the world. At last count the website listed fifty-seven separate trials involving yoga. Here's a partial list of the topics being studied:

- Effects of Yoga in Breast Cancer Patients
- Evaluation of Yoga for the Treatment of Pediatric Headaches
- A Study of Integrated Yoga Practice for Treating Geriatric Insomnia
- Yoga: Effect on Attention in Aging and Multiple Sclerosis
- Yoga for Treatment of Hot Flashes
- Yoga as a Treatment for Insomnia
- Yoga for Arthritis
- Yoga for Women Attempting Smoking Cessation
- Yoga for Patients with Epilepsy
- The Therapeutics Effects of Yoga in Individuals with Parkinson's Disease
- Evaluation of Multi-component Yoga Intervention as Adjunct to Psychiatric Treatment for Vietnam Veterans with Post Traumatic Stress Disorder (PTSD)
- Yoga Breath Program and Client-Centered Exposure for Relief of PTSD in Tsunami Victims

Who's Sari Now?

From one tiny Vancouver storefront to more than eighty retail out-
lets worldwide, athletic outfitter lululemon is one of the greatest
Canadian success stories of recent years. The high-profile brand has
enjoyed even more spectacular growth since going public in July
2007. Not bad for a company that does little advertising. Instead
lululemon relies on great word of mouth, spreading its message to
the tight-knit yoga and healthy-lifestyle communities through
"ambassadors," local athletes, instructors and others who "embody
the lululemon lifestyle." The company has also benefited from a
socially conscious and antiestablishment reputation, encapsulated
by the company's shaggy, feel-good manifesto. Among its maxims:
"Do one thing a day that scares you," "Success is determined by
how you handle setbacks" and "What we do to the earth we do to
ourselves."[33]

Consumers willing to pay a premium for high-tech sportswear
made from organic, renewable or just plain underused materials
were particularly attracted to the company's VitaSea clothing line.
Ranging in price from $50 to $120, VitaSea items were made up of
70 percent cotton, 6 percent spandex and 24 percent seaweed fiber,
which reduced stress and provided antibacterial, hydrating and
detoxifying benefits, according to lululemon. (You know yogis are
the target consumers when a retailer busts out the word *detoxifying*.)
According to clothing tags, the fabric released "marine amino acids,
minerals and vitamins into the skin upon contact with moisture."

But something about these seaweed shirts soon started to smell
fishy. It all started with the pesky *New York Times* and a November
2007 headline that said it all: " 'Seaweed' Clothing Has None, Tests
Show." Acting on a tip-off from a potential investor and evidently
doubting the whole VitaSea narrative, hard-nosed investigators from
the Gray Lady took the clothes down to the crime lab for analysis.
(Can anyone say "slow news day"?) Uh-oh. Two separate tests found
"no evidence of seaweed in the lululemon clothing," according to
the article. Dennis "Chip" Wilson, lululemon's founder, sputtered
out this response for the *Times*: "If you actually put it on and wear
it, it is different from cotton. That's my only test of it." It was not

good news for a company the *Times* described as having "found a lucrative niche selling athletic clothes wrapped in feel-good messages about friendship, love and life."[34]

The backlash was predictable: "lululemon just got a crash course in satya," a writer for the Montreal-based yoga magazine *ascent* posted to that magazine's website.[35] "It is about time all eco-retailers' products come under the same strict scrutiny that other retail businesses always have," a yogi wrote on the *Yoga Journal* blog.[36] Even a website billing itself as a simple tourist guide to Vancouver got dragged into the seaweed scuffle, setting up an insanely specific thread titled "Bad lululemon Experiences." "I will never buy Lulu again!" was one typically pithy post.[37]

Of course, the media also heaped scorn, Peter Foster of Canada's *Financial Post* being probably the most scabrous. In an article headlined "lululemon Asked for It," Foster wrote that the claims this "New Age yoga-wear peddler" made about VitaSea "rank up there with the alleged magic powers of rhinoceros horn, ursine penises and crystal pyramids." Foster then quoted a professor of nutritional sciences at the University of Toronto who described as laughable the notion that anything worthwhile could be absorbed from VitaSea clothing. Foster wasn't done: "lululemon isn't selling science, it's selling lifestyle and exclusivity, the chance to be on the environmentally aware inside, looking out at the tubby, Wal-Mart-shopping hoi polloi." What Foster found most grating was lululemon's manifesto, which pronounced "Coke, Pepsi and all other pops will be known as the cigarettes of the future" and declared colas were "just another cheap drug made to look great by advertising." "Such a statement should surely invite questions about expensive sportswear 'made to look great' by bogus marketing and junk science," Foster railed.[38] (Two months later, lululemon deleted its references to Coke and Pepsi. "We update the manifesto regularly in order to stay fresh in message," chief executive Bob Meers told the Canadian Press.)[39]

To stop the bleeding, lululemon moved fast. On the same day that Foster's article appeared, Canada's Competition Bureau, an independent law-enforcement and consumer-advocacy agency, announced that lululemon had agreed to remove all therapeutic and performance claims from its VitaSea clothing labels. That wasn't fast enough. The whole briny brouhaha had already brought to the surface other less-than-savory lululemon lore. It was revealed that the company that so often touts its commitment to local communities and so loudly proclaims its Vancouver roots had moved the bulk of its manufacturing offshore, from Canada to China, Taiwan, Indonesia and India. "Global economic forces ... have shifted manufacturing to more cost-attractive locations and resulted in closures of some domestic factories," the company's website states.[40] Also uncovered was the link between lululemon founder Wilson and Landmark Education Corp., a successor to est, or Erhard Seminars Training; est (like lululemon, always written lowercase), the confrontational human-potential movement of the seventies and eighties developed by former Scientologist Werner Erhard, included celebrities such as songwriter John Denver and actor Raul Julia among its devoted and vocal adherents. Yet there were enough psychotic episodes reported among other est attendees, according to a 1977 article in *The New York Times,* to prompt three psychiatrists "to alert their profession to the possibility that the experience may have devastating effects on some people."[41]

Critics are as wary of Landmark as they were of est, citing the company's own registration form as evidence of what the Landmark forum is capable of. Under the heading "Notice of Important Information, Health Warnings, and Legal Agreements," Landmark states a small fraction of attendees "have reported more serious symptoms ranging from mild psychotic behavior to psychosis occasionally requiring medical care and hospitalization" and that among a smaller group "there have been reports of unexplained suicide or other destructive behavior."[42] But Chip Wilson believes in Landmark's teaching seminars so wholeheartedly that lululemon foots the $495 fee for any employee who wants to attend. While Wilson has said the courses aren't a requirement, employees could be forgiven for thinking they're mandatory. In its 2007 Securities Registration Statement, a financial disclosure form required of any business offering securities in the United States, lululemon lists Landmark Education as required curriculum.

Six months after the initial flare-up, the Seaweed Scandal was a distant memory, especially where it mattered: Wall Street. "Profits soar at lululemon" the *Vancouver Sun* reported in April 2008 as the company "parlayed strong fourth-quarter sales into a quadrupling of profits.... The company expects 2008 revenues will range from about [Can]$370 million to $375 million."[43] It was also announced that lululemon's CEO during the Seaweed Scandal, Robert Meers, was being replaced by Christine Day, a former Starbucks senior manager and sales exec. All in all, "the numbers," as financial analyst Rick Aristotle Munarriz wrote on the *Fool.com* website, "prove that shoppers couldn't care less about the CEO's past or seaweed fiber's future."[44]

This is perhaps the most telling part of the Seaweed Scandal; the whole fishy flap crashed onshore with a roar yet ebbed away with a whisper. A brief paroxysm of blogging, some consternation, a little eye-rolling, and that was it. No boycotts, no burning the company's Deep V™ with iPod Shuffle pocket™ bra.

Dude, where's my outrage? Were yogis willing to accept this breach of satya just because it was wrapped up in the right robes? It's hard to tell the forced, phony benevolent enviro-hype from the naked rapacity nowadays, and it doesn't seem to make any difference anyway. It's brilliant, really. Corporations such as lululemon, having already appropriated everything, including rebellion, now hope we'll put our money where our distaste for materialism is. The last best hope today's flummoxed consumers have of registering their disapproval of consumer culture is by choosing high-priced consumer goods with the right "message."

In 2005 a brand-new word came into being, coined and defined by political satirist Stephen Colbert in October 2005 during the debut episode of his send-up of news shows, *The Colbert Report.* "Truthiness" is the "truth that comes from the gut, not books," the truth "one wishes to believe, rather than what is known to be true." *Truthiness* was subsequently voted the American Dialect Society and Merriam-Webster Word of the Year.

We yogis are struggling so much with satya. We confuse being truthful with knowing the Truth. We live in online echo chambers where we can block out every difficult or contrary opinion. We blurt out half-baked half-truths yet withhold our most sincere thoughts out of political correctness or fear of humiliation. Meanwhile, the lies, distortions and manipulations of modern life have rendered the truth all but unrecognizable anyway. We have witnessed the death of satya by a thousand deceits. So I would like to propose that yogis replace the pursuit of satya with the pursuit of Truthiness. The Truthiness is Out There, and it's so much easier to attain.

And if that doesn't work, let's just leave satya behind and move on. Asteya, the rejection of anything that's not rightfully ours—now there's a yama the yoga community can get behind!

9

Steal This Yoga

No one can get anything unless he earns it. This is
an eternal law.
—SWAMI VIVEKANANDA, *THE COMPLETE WORKS OF
SWAMI VIVEKANANDA*

I seem to be going in endless uphill loops. I'm on my way to meet the McCauleys, a self-described "yoga family," although I'm more than slightly lost as my car twists helplessly around this verdant, hilly patch of San Rafael, California. After a few more concentric circles I happen upon the house, perched on a tight corner and jutting out over the incline below. Vanessa Calder, one of six McCauley children who all do yoga, comes out to greet me. She's eight months pregnant, but not your typical eight months pregnant. With her wide smile, bouncy manner and blond hair pulled back neatly, she looks more like a teenager who just happens to be carrying a basketball than an expectant twentysomething. Her parents are still on their way from Sacramento, she tells me.

The inside of the house is airy and welcoming. Large windows look out onto tall trees, cloaking the house in scented shade. The signs of nesting are everywhere: in the half-finished baby's room, a new crib, various stuffed humanoid and mammalian toys, books dissecting the twin tumults of pregnancy and childrearing. The whole place feels very nurturing.

Bill and Sandy arrive. Bill is tall, tanned and tattooed, a long shock of graying hair topping his slender frame. An amulet hangs from a chain around his neck. This is how you might expect a professional surfer to age. He's sixty-two, he'll tell me later, but I'd believe fifty. His wife, Sandy (they met in college at the beginning of the sixties), looks just as youthful, maybe more so. She's trim and light on her feet, like him, and also spangled with jewelry. With her long black hair tumbling down her back and a shawl wrapped around her shoulders, she emits the bohemian gypsy-witchy vibe essentially trademarked by Stevie Nicks. They look good. They look happy. I realize then that the McCauleys are a myth come to life. They are the quintessence of California's bygone counterculture, an all-growed-up Age-of-Aquarius family living by an earthy play-together-stay-together ethos. (It could only happen here, in Marin County, a ground zero of natural beauty, liberal politics and affluence. Marin County has the highest per capita income in the United States, according to the last U.S. Census, in 2000.)

We sit down in the living room to talk. The genial patter and physical ease among the three makes conversation comfortable. There's no reserved paterfamilias, no sense of a domineering mother. Vanessa calls them Bill and Sandy. They laugh often. We begin to speak about things McCauley and yoga. Sandy found yoga in the early seventies, she tells me. "I ran an elementary school called the Sacramento Free School. All types of alternative people came there. This one woman taught me some yoga postures and I tried a few and they were, you know, marvelous," she says. "You start feeling the life force coming into your body and you start feeling a natural high."

Bill came to the practice through a more tortured route. He was a pre-med studying biology at the University of San Francisco in the sixties when the war in Vietnam began and he was called up for duty. He returned from the conflict a decorated infantry captain. He had a Bronze Star in his hand but an ache in his heart—a duality typical of the time. "With remorse for having been involved in an action designed to take life, the idea of enhancing and healing life had a great appeal to me," Bill writes in his teaching biography. He was soon spending time on all sorts of alternative pursuits, including yoga. "My first yoga teacher was eighty-five years old and we used to take private classes in her home. I was amazed at what wonderful shape this woman was in at eighty-five. I thought there was something here," he says.

I marvel inwardly again at Bill and Sandy's vibrancy. If naysayers still need proof of what yoga can do, I'm talking to it. They are the picture of perfect health. But it wasn't always the case. Around late 1992, at the age of forty-eight, Sandy had become decrepit, as she describes it. "I had enormous back pain, and I had gained a lot of weight." She tried acupuncture, went to a chiropractor, even considered back surgery. Eventually, she found another course: "I decided to just try yoga. So, I took up yoga on a daily basis for a year. Within three months, I already felt like a different person. But by the end of the year I had lost fifty pounds and my back pain was completely gone and I felt fabulous." Yoga, which had long been a *part* of her life, was about to *become* her life. Although she'd been practicing primarily Iyengar style, she'd also started going across the bridge to San Francisco three times a week to try another kind of yoga she found very therapeutic. One day in 1994 she saw a notice at the studio advertising a teacher-training conference. "And I thought, Wow, I'd really like to do that," she says. Sandy left Bill with their youngest daughter, Arbor, and went off for three months to Beverly Hills. It was the first formal teacher training that Bikram Choudhury had ever held.

Sandy returned from training trim, rejuvenated and refreshed—in turn getting Bill, son Mark, and daughters Arbor and Vanessa also interested in Bikram Yoga. "When I found out what yoga did for her [Sandy], I didn't need to know what it might do for me," Vanessa says. "I'm eight and a half months pregnant and don't have any back pain."[1] Soon after the Bikram training Sandy decided she wanted to open her own yoga studio. Bill was a licensed contractor and decided to build the studio himself, with help from Mark. Vanessa was studying business in New York when her mother called to announce that she was opening a yoga studio. "That scared me! She has incredible passion, incredible drive, amazing leadership skills, and communication skills and integrity, but not a lot of interest in keeping the books. So I came back, before I even started business school, to start the books," Vanessa explains. They christened the business "Yoga Loka."

Bill was feeling an itch. "I'd wanted to get out of the construction business for years," he says. Now he wanted a part of Sandy's yoga business. Fate intervened. "I cut my thumb off one day on the job. And I thought, This is a sign." He left the business in his son's hands and began teaching at Yoga Loka. When Sandy's father died, Bill and Sandy moved back to her hometown of Sacramento to be near Sandy's mother. There they opened another studio. A third studio soon followed. Long the bedrock of the McCauley marriage and the family's lifestyle, yoga had now become the cornerstone of a thriving family business.

But an egregious breach of yoga ethics was allegedly taking place inside Yoga Loka. The McCauleys claim that it was happening unknowingly, but it didn't matter. As quickly as the business had been built up, someone was now threatening to tear it down.

Thou Shalt Not Steal

In Sanskrit, the word *steya* means "robbery." Adding the prefix *a* to a word negates its meaning; thus *a-steya,* the third yoga yama, means abstention from theft or stealing. Of course, as with all the other yamas, this cursory definition fails to grasp the breadth of the meaning. Asteya also encompasses the notion of asceticism—taking only what one needs and no more. Ultimately, asteya means a freedom from desire, a state of mind in which there is absolutely no desire or impulse to take what is not ours. "That man has reached immortality who is disturbed by nothing material," as Swami Vivekananda once said.

Not surprisingly, the broader the definition, the harder asteya is to stick to. We steal so many things in so many ways that we've become almost blind to it; we cheat on our tax returns, we take welfare benefits we might not need, we stretch the truth on our insurance claims, we want a higher wage than our coworkers for the same work, we park in the handicapped zone when we're in a hurry. We steal intangible things too, such as control, attention or credit. We rob ourselves by neglecting our talents, by ignoring the chance to repair an ailment, by failing to do activities that rejuvenate and nourish us. All of these transgressions can also be seen as breaches of ahimsa, the underpinning of all yoga teachings. And stealing often requires deliberate falsehood, steering us back toward satya, truthfulness, the second yoga yama.

Stealing seems to be so firmly embedded in our lifestyle that you'd think some wiggle room might have developed here. But you'd be wrong. In our proprietary and possessive culture, asteya seems to be the one yama that the yoga industry has truly embraced, the one yoga edict that seems to have real meaning. Although it's not the part about renunciation or asceticism that we've taken to heart. Our version of asteya is much simpler and more narrowly focused. It usually goes something like this: Hands off my yoga!

Traditionally, the intricate techniques of yoga were passed down freely from teacher to student. The present-day yoga industry, in contrast, is an intellectual-property minefield. Ownership squabbles are constantly being fought over thousands of yoga styles that each represent a highly marketable intellectual commodity. And yogis who otherwise have little interaction with or inclination toward understanding the ethical underpinnings of yoga suddenly become indignant, screaming to the rooftops that each infraction is a slight against asteya.

By 2002 the McCauley family was running three studios in the San Francisco area, teaching primarily Bikram Yoga, the yoga Sandy had paid to learn at Bikram's teacher-training session. But the McCauleys weren't interested in being officially affiliated with Bikram's organization, the Yoga College of India. In particular, their son, Mark, had other ideas. He wanted to teach other yoga styles, maybe mix up the hot yoga series a little—freedoms prohibited under Bikram's affiliation guidelines. "He was a visionary. He wanted to move on with yoga, and that wouldn't be allowed with the Yoga College of India," Bill says about his son. "So, it was either us against our son, or the alternative. We love our son. We didn't want to stymie him or throw him out of the business, so we chose not to be a Yoga College of India." The next step was telling Bikram. That part didn't go so well. According to Sandy, Bikram "felt betrayed and angry. And we started feeling the repercussions."

Copyrighting Karma

The old days of the Bikram Yoga "affiliate" program were informal. With Bikram's permission and by agreeing to follow a few basic rules, recently certified teachers could either open their own studios or a Yoga College of India. But by 2002 much of the company's revenue was coming from teacher training, and the Bikram organization was in a franchising fury, with Yoga College CEO Leslie LaPage announcing aggressive plans to have "our yoga program and philosophy in every major city in the world."[2] Copyright protection was an important part of those plans. Bikram first applied for copyright protection in January 1979 for a book he'd published titled *Bikram's Beginning Yoga Class*. Over the years he filed additional copyrights for various books, audiotapes, videotapes and other Bikram Yoga products.

To really sell the franchise idea, it was thought, Bikram would need an "asset" to control. The answer came in 2002 when Bikram filed for copyright protection for the Bikram Yoga sequence itself, a move that shocked the yoga world. Filing the claim as an addendum to the existing copyright for his *Beginning Yoga Class* book, Bikram claimed that the new copyright gave him exclusive rights to the series. He also applied for trademark protection for the names Bikram Yoga, Bikram Hot Yoga, Bikram's Yoga College of India and Bikram's Beginning Class.

Rumors immediately began swirling that Bikram would aggressively pursue studios he thought weren't toeing the line. Bikram hired Akin Gump Strauss Hauer and Feld, one of the world's largest and most high-powered law firms, with over a thousand attorneys, advisers and lobbyists throughout North America, Europe and Asia. At the hands of Akin Gump lawyers, a comprehensive list of infractions became alleged copyright infringements overnight, including teaching without Bikram's accreditation, teaching variations of the Bikram series, teaching styles other than Bikram Yoga at a Bikram-affiliated studio and training teachers in the Bikram method. It all came to a head in June 2002 when Akin Gump sent more than fifty cease-and-desist letters to yoga studios across the United States and Canada, claiming they were in breach of Bikram's copyright and demanding that they stop teaching Bikram Yoga or face legal action. The letters claimed Bikram was entitled to "statutory damages of up to $150,000 per infringement."

Yoga Loka was among the studios to receive such a letter. Sandy McCauley was devastated. "What I saw it saying was 'Go out of business now, because you're not doing exactly what I want you to do,'" she says. "It scared me to death. It hit me in a place where my security was. We'd been in business for eight years or something and we were making our retirement on it, our family was involved and just the possibility of that collapsing was very frightening to me." For Bill the emotions were different. "It didn't bother me. I've been a warrior my whole life, I've been to war. This whole thing with Bikram didn't affect me," he says. But the legal facts remained, and none of the McCauleys knew quite what to do. "I'd never gotten a letter from an attorney before, a red letter from an attorney. It's definitely not something to be taken lightly. It's not something that you can ignore and hope that it goes away," Vanessa says. "We had to find a lawyer."

That's where Jim Harrison comes in. "I was getting into yoga; I was one of those people you see on the street carrying a pink yoga mat and coming out sweating and looking exhausted," says the husky, cheerful Harrison.[3] Having just finished studying law, Harrison was now studying yoga with Sandy and Bill McCauley. "I was starting a practice and trying to figure out how to get business and get my name around. And I said to them, 'Is there any kind of legal services that you need that we could exchange or trade for yoga?'" Harrison recalls. A few months later the cease-and-desist letter arrived. "Sandy McCauley comes to me holding this letter saying, What do I do?"

Harrison's first instinct was that the McCauleys band together with other studios under attack. "There was this body of people that were all saying the same thing and had the same fears and worries," Harrison says. "My advice to my client was to organize, put together an organization to provide a common voice and a pooling of resources." Harrison believed an umbrella organization would protect individual studio owners, what he refers to as safety in numbers: "We had all of these people scared to death of Bikram and his litigious nature. They didn't have the money to fight individually. They were all afraid of becoming targets individually." (*Mother Jones* magazine, in its reporting on the case, claimed some studio owners refused to discuss Bikram in print and were even afraid to identify themselves in telephone conference calls.)[4]

Harrison created a nonprofit legal entity and registered it with the state of California. He called the group Open Source Yoga Unity (OSYU), a name inspired by the Open Source software movement, which rejects intellectual property and ownership restrictions and holds that source code should be freely available for use and enhancement in the marketplace. "Rather than choosing to enforce rights to the source code they [Open Sourcers] release the code so that people can work with it, modify it, use it in their own products and continue it for the general good of the software programming community," explains technology journalist and *Eweek.com* news editor John Pallatto.[5] For Harrison the parallel between the yoga copyright case and the Open Source software movement was clear. "Yoga's been around thousands of years. It's developed, it's morphed. It's gone this direction and that direction. You add music, heat, meditation and it's constantly moving. If somebody controls a part of it, then its development in other directions could be hampered, prevented. That's just not right," he says.

I've spent the last few years of my life chasing yogis. By the time I met John Pallatto, he was something of a rare bird. "I have no personal interest in yoga. I don't practice yoga. My closest association with yoga is that my daughter occasionally attends yoga classes," he tells me. However, Pallatto was soon keeping an eagle eye on the OSYU case, intrigued by OSYU's approach of "taking on the mantle of Open Source software as their cry of liberty." OSYU soon set up a website. Boldly emblazoned on each page of the site was the group's mission: "To resist the enforcement of the copyright protection of any yoga style thereby ensuring its continued natural unfettered practice for all to enjoy and develop."[6]

Can any one individual really control yoga? Can something that never really belonged to anyone in the first place be stolen? To really grapple with the underlying issues the case raises, a dangerously rudimentary lesson in intellectual property law is in order. (These details relate to American law, although intellectual property laws are similar the world over.) The three pillars on which intellectual property law stands are patents, trademarks and copyright. A patent is the grant of a property right to an invention or process, excluding others from making, using or selling that invention or process. Trademark law protects definitive words, names, symbols, devices and the like that distinguish one provider of goods or services from another. Trademarks prevent others from using a confusingly similar mark but cannot prevent others from offering the same goods or services under a clearly different mark. Copyright law protects original works of authorship such as literary, dramatic, musical and visual works, both published and unpublished, that exist in some tangible medium such as a screenplay or website. An idea cannot be copyrighted, so copyright only protects the *form* of expression, not the subject matter. A specific description of a building can be copyrighted, but someone else can still write his or her original description of that same building and claim copyright on it. For an example of how these pillars relate to one another, consider a car manufacturing plant in, oh, say, Japan (Toyota City, to be exact). Patent law covers the unique assembly of cars at that plant. Trademark law covers the names "Toyota," "Prius," and so on. And copyright law covers the company's North American slogan "Toyota. Moving Forward."

Bikram's argument relies on copyright and, partly, trademark law. There's no argument about the validity of the copyright on Bikram's books, audiotapes or videos based on his series. Each of these works meets the requirement as an original work of authorship in a tangible form. It's the *scope* of protection these copyrights offer that's at issue. Does the protection extend to the series itself? Bikram says yes. OSYU disagrees. "He's doing something with copyright law that hasn't been done before, and he's really on shaky ground," says Jim Harrison. "If you can [copyright yoga], what protections do you have under it? We can't really walk away from this without that resolved one way or another."

Bikram isn't saying he owns or has control over any single yoga pose, poses that inarguably belong in the public domain. He's not

even saying he invented the hot and physical style he's become associated with. (After all, Bikram had to learn the ropes, too. His
teacher was the renowned Kolkata guru Bishnu Ghosh at the
College of Physical Education in Kolkata. Of course, Ghosh also
needed training. His guru was his older brother, Paramahansa
Yogananda, the prominent yogi who founded the Self-Realization
Fellowship in California. And let's not forget Yogananda had been
sent to America in 1920 by *his* teacher to spread the word of yoga
that had just been taught to him. And on and on it goes.) What
Bikram *is* claiming, however, is that by selecting twenty-six specific
postures and developing the sequence by adding two breathing exercises, the dialogue and the heat, he has created an original work of
authorship, in much the same way that a composer arranges existing
notes to create new music or a choreographer creates a new dance
from existing steps.

Jim Harrison rejects the choreography analogy because a yoga
sequence is not creative or expressive like dance but is instead functional, he says. "This is a sequence that was created for medical pur-
poses and not to 'say' anything," Harrison claims. "That's not what
copyright is meant to protect. If you come up with this great invention that has medical significance and you want to protect it, you
have to go to the patent office. He went to the wrong office." And
Bikram's claims that he has created something unique miss the larger
point, according to Harrison: "It's not the question of whether it's
unique but whether you can control a style of yoga. An analogy
would be if somebody in the Yankees pitching staff pitched a new
pitch and wrote about it and said, 'Okay, it's mine; you have to pay
me.' It starts to get absurd very quickly."

Elements of Bikram's argument do have merit. The copyrighted
Bikram dialogue is a (maddeningly) detailed description of how to
perform each pose in the Bikram Yoga series. The phrases will be
familiar to anyone who's ever set foot in a Bikram studio. "Bounce a
couple of times like a motorcycle ride," "your right leg should look
like a perfect upside-down L," "back, back, way back, fall back."
Bikram has accused nonlicensed teachers of using the dialogue
without his express permission, and he may have a case here, as
copyright also grants control over any public performance of copy-

righted material. Some studios may also violate Bikram's trademarks by using his name and logos without a license, although this issue is also a little more complicated than it might seem. Over time, the words *Bikram Yoga* have become almost synonymous with the concept of hot yoga. "Bikram Yoga is used to describe half the yoga conducted in a hot room. It does not necessarily mean that it is being provided to you only by Bikram's College of India," says Jim Harrison. Many people use the names interchangeably, without intending to violate Bikram's trademark. Like "aspirin," "hula hoop," "zipper" and "granola," the name Bikram Yoga is becoming generic. It's no longer a unique brand but the thing itself, in this case hot yoga. And when something becomes generic it's no longer entitled to trademark protection.

Om™

Despite what many legal industry experts considered a shaky claim at best, and considering the heavy hitters aligning against him, Bikram's cease-and-desist campaign was having success. A remarkable number of studios simply caved in to his demands and stopped teaching his series and using his name. But one studio hadn't buckled. Like Sandy McCauley, Kim Morrison had attended Bikram's first teacher-training program in 1994. Two years later she opened a studio in Costa Mesa, California, with her attorney husband, Mark, whom she trained to teach the Bikram series. (Similarly, Sandy and Bill had taught Vanessa how to teach the Bikram style.) When the studio wouldn't follow his demands, Bikram sued it in federal court. Open Source watched the case closely, hoping for legal direction.

It wasn't to be. In June 2002 the parties settled, with the Morrisons agreeing in part to no longer teach Bikram Yoga and to remove Bikram's registered trademarks from their studio, their advertising and all other printed materials. Bikram soon claimed the settlement as a victory. "Mr. Choudhury castigated the couple with the kind of grandiosity he is sometimes known for," a *New York Times* article asserted. "They are on the street today.... They are closing their school. They cannot say my name. She cannot teach my yoga anymore, because she lost her license," Bikram was quoted as

Intellectually Stimulating

The Bikram suit may have raised a giant stink within yoga circles, but it's just one case in the increasingly ludicrous world of intellectual property law. In 2006 *Mother Jones* uncovered some surprising facts about copyrights, trademarks and patents:

- Patent lawsuits in the United States have more than doubled since 1992.
- U.S. intellectual property is valued at $5.5 trillion, almost half the country's gross domestic product and greater than the GDP of any other nation but China.
- "Sensory Trademarks" include a duck quacking (AFLAC), a lion roaring (MGM), yodeling (Yahoo!) and giggling.
- Ninety-one pending trademarks bear Donald Trump's name, including "Donald J. Trump the Fragrance" and "Trump's Golden Lager." Not included is the phrase "You're fired."
- Martin Luther King Jr.'s estate charges academic authors $50 for each sentence of the "I Have a Dream" speech they reprint.
- Microsoft UK held a contest for the best film on intellectual property theft; finalists had to sign away all intellectual property rights on "terms acceptable to Microsoft."
- To prevent piracy of *Harry Potter and the Goblet of Fire,* a Montreal Cineplex monitored audiences with metal detectors and night-vision goggles and checked popcorn for video cameras.
- Nearly 20% of the 23,688 known human genes are patented in the United States. Private companies hold 63% of those patents.

saying. "That's why America is a great country. They have something called law and justice, and they use it."[7] For OSYU, the settlement was troubling. Without a ruling there was no clarification on the legal issues involved. "When it ended without clarification we kind of had a really important decision to make: Do we take the next step? What is the next step?" Vanessa Calder remembers thinking.

The whys, wherefores and whatnots of the case quickly engulfed its participants, as leading yogis and industry watchers staked out positions on both sides of the argument. Baron Baptiste briefly lived at Bikram's house while he studied the Bikram method and maintains a good relationship with Bikram, despite some ups and downs. He believes Bikram is well within his rights: "If Bikram wants to copyright his yoga series, this is America, and he has the right to copyright his yoga series. If it bothers you, well, look at yourself, not at Bikram." Baron's peer Rodney Yee couldn't disagree more about copyrighting a yoga sequence. "I could do it just to make money. I mean, really, it's just a money-making thing, right?" he asks. "I have no desire to do that. Zero desire. It's information. It comes and goes. It's alive." Tony Sanchez was a Bikram instructor until the two had a falling-out. On this issue he sides with his former guru. "If it is a system that your school is teaching that is very different from all the other systems, why shouldn't you have the right to own it and to present it according to what you see is fit?" Sanchez asks. Trisha Lamb takes a wider view: "Bikram has every right to try to do what he wishes with the particular style and dialogue that he teaches.... It is not in the spirit of traditional yoga. But this is the West."

It wasn't just theoretical arguments. There were emotional dust-ups as well. Before long, stories began surfacing of friendships sundered and businesses broken. Jeff Renfro is at the center of one such story. You may already be familiar with Renfro. He holds the world record for the longest scorpion pose performed on a surfboard (one hour, fourteen minutes and thirty-two seconds), an accomplishment he nailed during a San Francisco parade in 1998. San Franciscans might also remember Renfro for his former employee Hamlet, a sewer-sniffing pig that Renfro "employed" at Plug Busters, the plumbing company he operated. Hamlet's talent for locating underground pipes too deep for even electronic equipment to find had him in the sights of CNN, innumerable talk shows and even the *National Enquirer*. Since ditching the plumbing business in 2000, fifty-one-year-old Renfro has become better known for Funky Door Yoga, the four Bay Area yoga studios he runs. Hamlet is absent from the yoga scene. The day I visit Renfro's Berkeley studio a flotilla of French bulldogs is instead at the ready. (Well, splayed out and snoring anyway.)

The cute-as-hell mascots are just one aspect of Funky Door that puts it decidedly outside the Bikram norm, given the guru's notoriously strict guidelines for how to operate an affiliate studio. In contrast to the usually staid Bikram environment, large-scale caricatures cover the Funky Door walls and lobby, portraits of everyone from Bill Clinton to Bikram himself performing postures from the Bikram series, and all drawn by Jeff's talented artist father, Ed Renfro. Renfro the Younger admits Bikram wasn't at all sure about this particular studio. "He thinks that dogs do not belong in a yoga studio. He thinks the name Funky Door is crazy and stupid," Renfro says. "I just don't think my schools are exactly the image of what he had in mind."[8]

The two men are good friends, though, and it's not hard to imagine why Bikram might have a soft spot for Renfro. Like Bikram, Renfro jokes easily and often and is not given to overanalysis. As the three of us settle down to talk turkey, I suspect we won't be spending too much time agonizing over breaches of asteya or compiling a dossier of non-yogic behavior. Don't get me wrong, Renfro knows what he feels and is quick to jump to Bikram's defense. He believes the guru has every right to protect the unique brand he has developed. "Bikram worked very hard all his life to get where he is," Renfro says. "What he's trying to do is keep his yoga pure so that when you call something Bikram Yoga you know he's teaching his yoga as it's meant to be taught."

This puts Renfro at odds with his old friend James Barkan, whose relationship with Bikram goes back much farther than Renfro's. The pair met in 1980 in Los Angeles, where Barkan had landed in pursuit of an acting and music career. Bikram took him under his wing, training him at the yoga master's Los Angeles headquarters, an intense experience that Barkan remembers fondly. "I was very inspired by Bikram's passion," he says. "He inspired me to do as much yoga as I could. We were fanatics, two or three of us; we did four to five yoga classes a day for two years."

By 1983 Barkan had ditched singing and acting and had returned to his native Florida to open his own Yoga College of India. Although rooted in the Ghosh lineage that inspired Bikram's series, Barkan's rigorous physical style has evolved. And that's exactly how it should be, he says. "The postures that are in Bikram's sequence ... are not Bikram's postures. They're postures that have been passed down from his teacher to his teacher, which Bikram passed to me. And I pass them to my students, which I believe is how the universe works." Jeff Renfro sees it differently: "If you're going to call it Bikram Yoga or give people the impression that it's Bikram Yoga, then it should be Bikram Yoga. I don't have the right to publish a song like 'It's a Hard Day's Night' by the Beatles, change two words and then make money off it." Barkan retorts, "It's not anyone's property to own, let alone to steal." And so on and so on.

By 2002 Barkan was training and certifying instructors to teach "Hot Yoga with Jimmy Barkan" (later to become the Barkan Method). By 2003 Barkan had signed on with OSYU in its suit against Bikram. Although he never received a cease-and-desist letter, Barkan had heard enough horror stories and decided a proactive approach was best. "I was just being offensive," he says with the hint of a grin. Barkan's move did not sit well with Jeff Renfro. "Some of the people who are suing Bikram are making a lot of money off changing the yoga a little bit. They have financial incentives for what they are doing," he says. Barkan is equally adamant that what he offers is unique. "I don't teach Bikram Yoga anymore. I teach 'Hot Yoga with Jimmy Barkan.'" To Bikram supporters, that's a distinction without a difference. Certainly it does highlight one of the more absurd aspects of the case—that it's essentially a semantic brouhaha. Simply change the name of your studio and you're off the hook. Sever your ties to Bikram and you will be set free. What has generated so much heartache among studio owners, however, is the belief that Bikram is *forcing* them to sever those ties. "I was Bikram's senior teacher. That's what he called me for fifteen years," says Barkan. "Because I'm now not playing the franchise game that Bikram wants everyone to play, then what? I should just stop teaching yoga altogether? Just stop helping people? No more helping people? Sorry."

Again, Jeff Renfro disagrees. "My name is a little bit odd to Bikram, the colors I paint here. He doesn't understand that I have dogs in my studio.... We don't have a lawsuit against each other," says Jeff Renfro. "If you're going to teach Bikram Yoga and use his name, he wants you to adhere to his rules and that I totally honor and understand. But at the same time, the way he's going about enforcing it is very fascist. The way he's going [about it] is very cruel sometimes," Barkan says. Jeff Renfro responds again. "Like all of us, his [Bikram's] bark is a lot worse than his bite. I think he just wants everybody to be happy and get along," he says. And so on and so on.

"It's unfortunate that this disruption in the yoga community has to take place. It's unfortunate that business has to intersect, but it is big business," says Jim Harrison. On this one point Team Bikram and Team Freedom can agree. "I think it's a very painful case. A lot of these people were very close to Bikram at one time," Jeff Renfro concedes.

For Vanessa, Bill and Sandy, the stakes aren't theoretical, they are real—and Sandy's frustration with the situation is becoming ever more apparent. "We're certainly not against Bikram. We like the yoga. We paid a good penny to take the training, and I just don't want to give it up," she says. Bill takes her hand. "All yoga is good yoga," he says. "The only bad yoga is saying that your yoga is the best or the only."

James Barkan shows me a photo of Bikram with his arms wrapped around Barkan's late father. "Nobody had a connection with Bikram more than I did.... We were very, very close. Our families were very, very close," he says. "We called each other brothers." I remind him that Bikram now calls people who teach similar styles to his "imposters" who "must and will be stopped." Barkan sighs. "I don't consider myself an imposter."

The question of whether someone can control yoga was looking as if it would indeed be settled in that most American of ways—in court. In December 2003 OSYU fired back at Bikram, filing an abuse-of-copyright claim against him for allegedly attempting to obtain a monopoly on teaching the Bikram Yoga series. In an even more audacious step, OSYU also asked a federal court for a declaratory judgment. Common in intellectual property litigation, a declaratory judgment states the rights, duties and obligations of each party regarding a disputed area of law without ordering any action or awarding any damages. OSYU hoped a federal judge would declare Bikram's claimed copyright and trademark as unenforceable, thereby ending the whole free-for-all. The request for judgment had an added strategic advantage: It turned Bikram the plaintiff into Bikram the defendant. Serving Bikram's lawyers the lawsuit, Jim Harrison says, was "like taking a stick to a beehive."

The case was becoming a legal cause célèbre, even attracting the interest of Stanford Law School professor Lawrence Lessig, described by *New York* magazine as "the most important next-wave thinker on intellectual property."[9] Lessig founded both Stanford's Center for Internet and Society and the copyright-system alternative Creative Commons and serves as a board member on the Electronic Frontier Foundation as well as on the Software Freedom Law Center. Intrigued by the case, Lessig offered OSYU some Center for Internet and Society services at no cost. (The judge assigned to the case, Phyllis Hamilton, of the Northern District of California, also happened to be a Stanford alumna.) "All of a sudden I have a number of attorneys who are seeing this as an exciting and interesting case for two reasons. One, they think that Bikram doesn't have a leg to stand on the copyright. And two, they like yoga, do it themselves and don't want to see anyone control it," Harrison says.

As rancorous as the situation had become, and as difficult as industry watchers find it to fathom, many studio owners in the OSYU camp maintain their respect for Bikram. Outsiders love to throw around words such as *thuggish* and *strong arm*, intimating Bikram is behaving like a gangster. OSYU members who know Bikram, meanwhile, seem to have adopted Michael Corleone's credo from *The Godfather*: "It's not personal, Sonny. It's strictly business." "I still have a very, very warm place in my heart for Bikram, even though we had political and business fallout. He's still family," James Barkan says. Despite that they no longer speak, Sandy McCauley says she still loves Bikram, "and always will, because I deeply appreciate what I gained in the training. It gave me the opportunity of awakening, truly being an awakened human being." Sandy's daughter Vanessa, who's never had a personal relationship with Bikram, takes the toughest stance toward him. "He has this wonderfully charismatic, flamboyant, exaggerated character. He says things that are fun, that are intense, that are sometimes appalling.… What becomes intolerable is when you take that flamboyance and attempt to enforce it by letter or law," she says. "This is our business. This is our livelihood. We don't want to see it destroyed by anybody, especially by somebody who we feel is acting in an unlawful way."

Patently Absurd

Perhaps it was inevitable that the ethical divide the Bikram case opened up would fester into an ugly ideological gash. The yoga community had long been riven by arguments over legally enforced ownership and entitlement. Into this tinderbox came Bikram, the perfect flashpoint. "It is not in any way surprising to me that someone copyrighted this and branded it and called it their own," says Stefanie Syman, author of *Practice: A History of Yoga in America.* "It's taking the business of yoga to its logical conclusion," she says. This perceived over-reliance on copyright is now one of the chief complaints (among a litany) leveled against today's yoga scene. Are these gurus really going to court to protect their yoga styles, or are they just trying to squeeze a(nother) buck out of hapless yogis? Industry watchers such as *Eweek.com* technology editor John Pallatto are skeptical. "It's sort of ironic that they [litigant yogis] are going against this philosophy and way of life that tries to assert a sense of inner peace and balance," he says. "It's clear that business is business and competition is competition, no matter whether you're selling software or philosophy or fitness."

Of course, Bikram isn't the only yogi who believes the levers of justice are there to keep sticky fingers away from his yoga. Long ago, the founders of yoga lineages such as Kundalini and Iyengar copyrighted their names, studios, books and videos and trademarked their logos and looks. It's all part of the decades-long battle among modern gurus to distinguish themselves from one another, says renowned yogi David Life, cofounder of the Jivamukti Yoga Center in New York. "There are Iyengar centers worldwide that have existed for dozens of years, Sivananda centers worldwide that have existed for twenty or thirty years; there are

Integral yoga centers worldwide," he tells me during a break at a yoga conference in New York. "When they [critics] talk about yoga franchises, of course, they don't talk about that."

While Jivamukti doesn't call itself a franchise, it certainly operates like one, keeping its licensed instructors and studio owners on a tight leash. It begins before teacher training, when all prospective Jivamukti teachers are asked to sign a teacher certification agreement. Considered fairly typical by industry standards, the Jivamukti agreement states that instructors may "not use, nor permit to be used, the words 'Jivamukti' and/or 'Jivamukti Yoga' in connection with any location other than an authorized Jivamukti Center ('JYC')."[10] The agreement also reminds instructors that "acceptance into the JYC partnership/licensing program is at the sole discretion of JYC." David Life has, in the past, supported Bikram's attempt to protect his sequence. "He can't let people run rampant with his name or distort it in any way they feel like on a whim," Life told *Yoga Journal* in 2003. "I totally understand where he's coming from. He's in a corner."[11] Life should know. He claims his Jivamukti method, too, has been stolen.

To a Sanskrit speaker, a *jiva mukti* is someone who is spiritually liberated and lives to benefit the lives of others. To yogis and just about anyone else within stone's throw of a farmers' market, Jivamukti is a powerful brand that conjures up images of Gwyneth Paltrow in eagle pose or Christy Turlington in downward dog. (To be sure, there are worse images to carry around in your head.) To David Life and cofounder Sharon Gannon, Jivamukti is a community that represents years of dedication, painstaking development and plain old hard work. Success has many fathers, it seems. In 2002 Life complained to *Business 2.0* magazine that his high-wattage clients were being lured away by Jivamukti-certified teachers who were opening up studios nearby. "They're not calling themselves Jivamukti, but the staff is almost 100 percent certified through our training program," Life was quoted as saying.[12] (Of course, they couldn't call themselves Jivamukti. As *Business 2.0* duly noted, that name is trademarked.)

Now I don't for a second doubt that Life's vegan heart is anything but pure. While most North American yoga schools play dumb when it comes to the yamas, Jivamukti makes a real effort to keep ethical concerns and social awareness front and center, especially the teaching of ahimsa, nonviolence toward oneself and others. Life and Gannon are both vocal animal rights activists. They regularly host benefits for animal, environmental and human rights causes. And in May 2006 Jivamukti opened a new Manhattan studio featuring reused furniture, nontoxic building materials and floor padding made from recycled car tires.

Gannon and Life may value ahimsa highly, but is it at the expense of asteya? Just over two years earlier, Life had been complaining that teachers were stealing his clients, yet his new studio happens to be in the same building as a successful and established Bikram Yoga studio. This is the studio where I used to practice, and I have to admit it saddens me to hear stories and read blogs about the effects of this sudden and stiff competition. "I remember rushing to a 5:30 P.M. class and cramming myself into the elevator with other students clutching their yoga mats," one Bikram yogi blogged. "I thought we were all rushing to class but did not realize that everyone except me was getting off on the second floor for their favorite Jivamukti class." To make matters worse, some of Jivamukti's best-known boldfaced benefactors are often seen bypassing Bikram. "Russell Simmons was on the elevator," the Bikram yogi blogged. "He kept staring at me, probably … baffled as to why I was not getting off the elevator with the rest of his yogi groupies."[13] I wonder if stealing someone's thunder counts as a breach of asteya?

With the previous two yamas, ahimsa and satya, it's our selectivity that causes problems; we proclaim strict adherence to ethical dictates that we ignore or bend when needed. With asteya the offense is believing *too much*. Present-day yogis believe so strongly in the cherry-picked definition that others shouldn't "steal" from them that they've gobbled up the rights to practically every yogic concept that can be legally pinned down. Nowadays you would be hard-pressed to find even a vaguely Eastern concept that's still in that quaint little corner we call the public domain. There's the prana (in Sanskrit, "life energy") clothing line, the Yoga Sutra ("lifeline") teacher-teaching program and the Om (a sacred Hindu, Jain and Buddhist utterance) series of videos, book and CDs. And don't forget the Patanjali, Asana and Ashtanga branded yoga styles. But be careful. While ashtanga translates literally as "eight limbs," Ashtanga yoga the *business* should not be confused with Eight Limbs Yoga, or even 8 Limbs Yoga (with a numerical "8," you see). It's so easy to get confused. There's a Yama yoga studio, a Yama Yoga studio and a Yoga Yama studio, as well as a Yama Yoga Center. One dash in the wrong place and you could easily have a civil suit on your hands. The overall impression is of an industry blissfully ignorant of its own rapaciousness and double standards. Do you suppose this is really what the founders of these great lineages had in mind?

It's irrational to pretend yoga can survive without competing in the global marketplace. At the same time, we must also recognize that branding serves a useful purpose. Brand recognition drives quality. With a recognizable yoga brand there is incentive to maintain a high standard, thus guiding customers toward a reliable source of good yoga. The question is, How do we strike a balance between modesty and market advantage? How can a yoga brand keep its stated aims in perspective (no more "shortcuts to Nirvana") without straying too far from the actual practice of yoga?

John Friend founded Anusara yoga (*anusara* means "flowing with grace" in Sanskrit) when it became clear he had strayed significantly from his Iyengar-style roots. The result is what *Yoga Journal* calls a quintessentially American yoga style. "It's upbeat, optimistic, entrepreneurial, systematic, and do-it-yourself-friendly, and it has elements of a quick fix. It's spiritual but not dogmatic," the magazine cooed, adding that Friend has created "a framework in which the less-exercised limbs of yoga—pranayama, meditation, philosophy, ethical precepts—can move about freely."[14] Friend has, of course, trademarked his style, believing that every yogi has the right to do so, "if you have some methodology that you feel is very specific and it has benefit and you feel that other people are gaining from that specific method."

In person Friend is low-key and open, traits reflected in the way he discusses and promotes his work. There's less hard sell in the Anusara world than with many other yoga styles; Friend and his practitioners rely instead on the notion that the yoga will sell itself.

Nor does Friend ask his instructors for a franchise fee. But he does expect his teachers to regularly reinforce where the style comes from, in this case from Iyengar and through Friend himself. This way, the yoga is never able to stray far from its roots in a venerable tradition. "I think the practitioner should honor the source. To take it and say 'It's mine,' well, that's not true. The truth is, you got it from this guy," Friend says. "That's Dharmic, that's proper." In fact, to snub the source, to withhold recognition that is not yours, is itself a breach of asteya, Friend reminds me. "When you don't give credit where credit is due you create an a-Dharmic situation."

Dharmic or not, this whole state of affairs looks pretty ridiculous when seen through the eyes of the dedicated Indian yogi. Many Indian practitioners view Western gurus as little more than thieves. Before anyone even thought of outsourcing, India's expat gurus were teaming up with Western entrepreneurs to tap India's vast traditional knowledge base of spiritual and physical healing for consumption in the West. By 2007 the U.S. government had issued 150 yoga-related copyrights, 134 patents on yoga accessories and 2315 yoga trademarks.[15]

In 2005 the Indian government fought back. At a press conference in the Indian capital of Delhi, Indian science and technology minister Kapil Sibal unveiled plans for a strange document aimed at fighting off the culture vultures. The Traditional Knowledge Digital Library, or TKDL, is an online database, just now in its infancy, that illustrates how hundreds of yoga postures, body-cleansing routines, ayurvedic remedies and other esoteric practices developed in India. Using the TKDL as proof that these practices are in that country's "cultural domain," the Indian government wants to reclaim its rights over them—not to mention the revenue made from the practices. "We want to completely patent our age-old methods and techniques to protect them. We have to protect our traditions and our database," said Sibal.[16]

The media were dubious, to say the least. They were stuck on how the TKDL would *work* exactly. The idea is this: Data are translated from ancient Sanskrit and Tamil texts, stored digitally in the database and made available, in five international languages, to groups such as the World Trade Organization and patent offices worldwide. The aim is for the TKDL to work as a sort of guidebook of traditional Indian practices. The hope, one assumes, is that patent issuers will realize that yoga wasn't created in southern California sometime in 1965.

While many people scratched their heads, there was little denying that the Indian government had a legitimate beef. Until now, Indians had just stood by and watched as westerners appropriated ideas as intrinsic to their culture as the Kama Sutra, one of India's most renowned texts that has now morphed magically into an online merchant flogging trinkets that "help loving couples enjoy intimacy."[17] Similarly, it must surely be unsettling to Indian traditionalists that a web search for "Mahatma" returns references to "America's favorite rice." "Should an Indian, in retaliation, patent the Heimlich maneuver, so that he can collect every time a waiter saves a customer from choking on a fishbone?" Indian novelist Suketu Mehta fumed in a *New York Times* op-ed piece.[18]

Come on now. That would be absurd.

10

Om for Wayward Boys

Chastity is the basis of all religions.
—SWAMI VIVEKANANDA, *THE COMPLETE WORKS OF
SWAMI VIVEKANANDA*

I've decided to visit a famous ashram. This isn't one of those run-of-
the-mill ashrams that dotted the North American landscape during
the seventies, the kind that exist now, if at all, as mere ghosts of their
former selves. This ashram is as influential today as it was during its
seventies heyday, the locus of a robust, worldwide spiritual movement that shows no sign of waning. This ashram has been credited
with everything from the time-honored turning-around-of-lives to
boosting the sagging economy of the once-tattered community it
now anchors.

Most important, the ashram has been home to two entrancing
and powerful gurus. The first was Swami Muktananda, an Indian
sage who came west in the seventies armed with an interpretation of
yoga that made him one of the world's most prominent and notorious mystical leaders. The second is the ashram's current spiritual
head, Gurumayi, a woman of such grace, such charisma, such beauty
that it's said followers are brought to tears, rendered speechless in her
presence. Yet for all her power, Gurumayi's public appearances have
become, for her loyal acolytes at least, distressingly rare. Most

ashram outsiders haven't seen her in more than four years. Her annual New Year's Day message, the cornerstone of her yearly philosophical rationing, used to be delivered in person. It's now prerecorded and delivered via video. And don't expect to see or read much about her in the media. Gurumayi doesn't give interviews. Nobody from the ashram does.

Well, maybe I can change all that, I figure, as I approach the main ashram entrance, an ornate welcoming arch with the phrase *see God in each other* carved into it. Now that I'm here it can't hurt to ask for an interview. Perhaps I'll nail a sit-down with a reclusive and bewitching spiritual titan. Maybe I'll get palmed off onto some PR flak. All they can do is say no.

I don't get past the front gate. A pathologically polite young man (monk? guard?) stationed at the arch informs me that, apparently, I don't have all the facts at my disposal. The ashram, which once welcomed pilgrims with open arms, no longer receives drop-in visitors, and that includes curious writers. (In 2004 the ashram board of trustees designated it as a place for "long-term retreat" only, later research reveals.)[1]

What a shame, I think to myself as I walk away. All those inaccessibly beautiful rolling hills, all that ornate and out-of-reach harmony. Is that much seclusion and foreboding really necessary to reach enlightenment? Come to think of it, *ashram* hardly seems the right word for this place. Fortress might be more apt. Or compound, the way that tiny slip of Hyannis Port where the Kennedys frolic is always called a compound, as if the people inside are far too valuable, or vulnerable, to interact with.

As I make my way back to my car I take one more look over my shoulder. This really is for the best I decide, considering how many stories I've heard about people who have entered this place never to return, not whole anyway. Then I pat myself on the back. I've gotten away. Not everybody escapes a guru's clutches so easily.

The guru-gone-bad is perhaps the most unsettling phenomenon in yoga's long and fascinating history. It's certainly one of the most frequent. And when the all-too-human desires of our Enlightened Ones break loose, when the pedestal finally topples, the results are often spectacularly scandalous. These eruptions take many forms—ethical mischief, political high jinks, financial shenanigans—although it's the outrages associated with the pleasures of the flesh that really get our blood boiling. For seekers this is where their immature desire to be coddled by an authority figure meets their very adult, sometimes very complicated, ideas about sexuality and social mores. For teachers, too, it's a minefield. In no other arena are their proclamations and promises under the microscope as they are with regard to their sex lives. We love playing "gotcha" with our gurus. And the gurus never seem to disappoint.

Thou Shalt Not Lust

The root word of *brahmacharya,* the fourth of the five yoga yamas, is *brahma,* the Sanskrit word for "deity." *Char,* the Sanskrit word for "walk," and *ya,* which means "actively," when paired together (*charya*) are most often translated as "practice." Thus, the literal translation of *brahmacharya* is "walking with God." It's come to mean self-control or chastity, specifically as an abstention from sensual indulgence, which can encompass everything from overeating to money hoarding.

A narrower translation of *brahmacharya* is celibacy or right sexual conduct. Although this is the most difficult definition for many westerners to understand, it's also the most common. (Something to do with our puritanical need to punish ourselves, I suspect.) For ascetic purists, such as the monks and nuns whose sexuality is consecrated to God, brahmacharya means complete abstention from sexual intercourse. Most present-day yogis interpret brahmacharya more as a restraint on meaningless sexual encounters, which might mean respecting our sexual partners, not using others solely for sex, remaining faithful within a monogamous relationship, and so on. Either way, for the purist or the modernist, the end result is supposed to be the same: We are to redirect our sexual energy toward devotion to God.

The edict of brahmacharya, no matter how you slice it, has been broken so many times that it's become a grand cliché. The oversexed guru romping with his doe-eyed followers has been a cultural touchstone since at least the late sixties, when John Lennon penned "Sexy

Sadie," a song about the Beatles' former guru, Maharishi Mahesh Yogi. (The song's original title was "Maharishi.") Lennon believed the guru's celibacy was a lie and suspected Maharishi had been sleeping with young women at his ashram. Since then, countless swamis have come unstuck, leading to endless newspaper exposés and tongue-in-cheek magazine articles questioning the very essence of the guru role. The depiction of holy man turned lascivious Lothario has become such a sore point that many traditional Hindus protested Mike Myers' 2008 film *The Love Guru* before it even came out. A self-described "Hindu leader" from Nevada feared the film, billed as a comedy about an oversexed and overly ambitious American-born guru, would do yet more damage to the already-battered guru brand and demanded that the studio releasing the film screen it for members of the Hindu community before its release. Studio officials agreed but not before pointing out that the film, hardly a trove of theological wisdom anyway, was a "nondenominational comedy" and that the character had his own "fictional belief system."[2] (This may leave the secularists among us questioning which religious belief system isn't fictional.)

Of course, most clichés form around a kernel of truth, and in this case it's a large kernel. Nobody denies that sexual transgressions are and have been rampant in the yoga industry. "Yes, it happens. It happens across all dimensions of human society. It happens among yoga teachers. It happens with Christian preachers. It happens all across society," says Trisha Lamb, former head of the California-based Yoga Research and Education Center. She doesn't believe these situations make any ultimate statement about yoga and instead feels the issue has been blown out of proportion. "The press loves sex scandals. They give them an inordinate amount of press. It makes it seem like the problem is all-pervasive in the yoga community, and it's not the case at all," she says.

The media have covered some of these scandals excessively and without much regard for perspective, but the reason for that is simple: They're cheap and easy stories to cover, and readers have lots of fun devouring them. Besides, just because a story appeals to our prurient instincts doesn't mean it's without value. On the contrary, some of these flameouts have been so fantastic and so revealing that the yoga industry would be unwise to ignore the issues that underlie them.

Transcendental Gratification

Twin desires ruled Amrit Desai's early life: yoga and the dream to come to America. Access to yoga proved no problem. Living in the tiny Indian village of Halol, Desai was introduced at age fifteen to the famed Indian yogi Swami Kripalvananda. Desai soon became his number-one student. Getting himself to the land of opportunity would prove more difficult for Desai. "I was fascinated by everything I had heard about America," he says. "It just, like, drew me." He eventually found a way to fulfill his dream. In 1960, at age twenty-eight, he applied to the Philadelphia College of Art and was accepted. "My real dedication and interest was yoga and a spiritual way of developing myself, but it was the only way I could come to America," he explains. It wasn't long before his true calling emerged. Within a month and a half he was teaching yoga.

Desai's small Philadelphia following grew rapidly. In 1966 Desai and nine followers formed the Yoga Society of Pennsylvania, hoping to spread the science and philosophy of yoga and to train Americans as teachers. By 1972 Desai, now also known as Gurudev, meaning "beloved teacher," felt he had become overly busy and decided to purchase a large property some thirty miles from Philadelphia with the intention of going on retreat there. But his followers didn't want to lose him. "Some of the advanced students, they said … 'We would like to continue studying with you and maybe live near you and help you do the gardening and shopping and everything,'" Desai recalls. Thus, the ashram began. "It just, like, grew out of my desire to move away from the hustle and bustle of the city and yoga classes. But they followed me!"

The numbers soon swelled. "Everywhere I went people would follow. They said, 'We want to be in your ashram,'" Desai says. In 1974 the nonprofit Yoga Society had changed its name to the Kripalu Yoga Fellowship. A year later, and with over fifty resident practitioners, the organization purchased a second and significantly larger facility where it could offer housing, group yoga instruction and meals—a complete immersion in the Kripalu experience.

Enthusiastic volunteers ran the facility, receiving a small stipend of $30 a month to cover personal items. (Volunteers were not salaried and therefore did not qualify for social security benefits.) Yogi Desai, the ashram's beloved leader and guru, received a wage for his spiritual guidance.

The energy at the ashram was, by all accounts, intense. Anne Simpkinson, former editor of the now defunct *Common Boundary* magazine, wrote in the excellent 1996 article "Soul Betrayal" that it was not uncommon for early ashramites "to have strong *shakti* (energy) experiences, such as automatic movement and writing, speaking in tongues, and sharp increases in body temperature. These experiences in part solidified Desai's guru status among many of his students; some disciples took them to mean that the guru must be bona fide and therefore infallible. For too many devotees this reasoning translated as giving over their sense of judgment in major life decisions."[3]

By the early eighties the Pennsylvania ashram was bursting at the seams. So in 1983 the group purchased a former Jesuit seminary in Massachusetts and opened the Kripalu Center for Yoga and Health. The organization remains there today. With over three hundred residents, it had become the largest yoga ashram in the United States, described in a 1989 *Hinduism Today* article as "a cyclone of activity and stillness."[4] By this time Kripalu had also slowly begun to merge traditional yoga beliefs with more New Age ideas about psychology and self-development. The organization was also asking more of its residents, who were 60 percent female, 40 percent male, mostly single and all volunteers. According to the Kripalu version of its history, posted on the group's website, ashram residents were being asked to take "formal vows of celibacy, obedience, and simplicity to declare their status as yoga monks and nuns."[5] It was classic brahmacharya. Yogi Desai, who was married with three children, told *Hinduism Today* how men and women lived separately, ate in different halls and traveled in separate cars. Yogi Desai believed celibacy was the key to much of Kripalu's success. Alas, celibacy would also propel Desai's own fall from grace.

Good Vibrations

"I never would have said Kripalu was a cult," one Kripalu yoga teacher says about the organization under Amrit Desai's leadership, "but now I understand that for people who lived there and were young and vulnerable, they were in a kind of trance. They gave over their lives in a way that is the hallmark of cults."

Awkward Positions

To many yogis, the idea of enforced celibacy raises more questions than it answers (eugenics, anyone?). Is sexual activity counterproductive to one's spiritual progress? Can't sex ever be a positive experience that moves us *toward* a spiritual goal? The implementation of such a policy also raises questions: Is the average ashramite, even those ignorant of yoga's ethical precepts, considered a true yogi only after he or she has given up sex? What about all those people who came to yoga already in a sexual relationship? And who's going to break the bad news to all those horny young men coming to yoga classes because they're jam-packed with hot chicks?

The easy way around these tricky questions is to enforce brahmacharya selectively—which is apparently what Yogi Desai did. Around 1986 a female devotee revealed she'd had a sexual relationship with Desai. He flatly denied the accusation, the community stood behind its guru and the woman left the ashram. End of story, so it seemed. The woman was vindicated eight years later, when another woman came forward to describe how she'd also had a sexual relationship with Desai. As more details emerged it was clear that the jig was up. Eventually, in an audiotaped statement, Desai admitted to sexual encounters with three female followers—all while preaching celibacy.

The scandal set off massive shock waves. The ashram began to crumble. Two-thirds of its residents fled, with more than one hundred former residents later filing a class-action lawsuit against the Kripalu Center. The management structure of the whole organization was turned upside down. And the organization found itself hundreds of thousands of dollars in debt. (The financial realities at Kripalu also came as a surprise to many long-term residents. Although top-level stipends were no more than $3400 a year, the organization paid Desai $155,000 annually. He also earned royalties from the sale of books and tapes.) Yet what upset ashramites was not dollars or dalliances, according to Anne Simpkinson. It was the deception. "What devastated many of Desai's followers far more than the revelations of his inappropriate sexual relations was the fact that he had hidden them and lied about them for so long," she wrote in the "Soul Betrayal" article. For their part, Kripalu's board of trustees, having confirmed the accusations against Desai, had little choice but to end its "contractual agreement" with him. The board asked him to resign. He agreed. By October 1994 Yogi Desai was no longer part of the organization he'd created.

Kripalu soldiered on, shedding its traditional guru-disciple structure and reforming as an essentially secular organization. In 1999 Kripalu officially stopped being a "religious order" and became a nonprofit "education and wellness center." The small but hardy band of residents who had weathered the storm went on to become paid employees. Today, Kripalu looks nothing like an ashram. It instead resembles one of those countless high-end day spas dotted across North America that offer respite to detoxing B-list celebrities and the stressed-out spouses of high-profile CEOs.

Desai's life and career continued as well. After a period of reflection, he opened the Amrit Yoga Institute and retreat center, housed on a secluded six-acre property in Salt Springs, Florida. He now teaches a style of yoga called the Amrit Method that the institute says evolved from the Kripalu method.

That's the conventional wisdom, anyway. I've arranged to meet Yogi Desai at a Zen Center in Rhode Island, about two hours due east of Kripalu headquarters, where he's conducting teacher training. I'm hoping to get Desai's side of the story, which has never really been told, although I've already been informed that questions about his ouster from Kripalu are off the table. (Legal proceedings, confidentiality, etc.) So I've made it clear to Malay, my main contact and Yogi

Desai's son, that I'd like to discuss the guru-disciple relationship in depth, as a backdoor way to perhaps uncover some new nugget about the Kripalu story.

I arrive at the Zen Center a day ahead of our scheduled interview in order to meet Yogi Desai, to perhaps interview some of his followers and maybe even squeeze in a yoga class or two. Malay leads me through to Yogi Desai's room. It's monastic at best: a small bed next to a tiny cupboard and sideboard. Yogi Desai stands to greet me. He's tall and spry with a wide, warm smile. He takes my hand and we talk trivialities for a while (traffic, the view out his window). He says he's thinking of taking a nap, so I leave him in peace. Later that evening, during a yoga class, Desai calls me to the front of the auditorium and introduces me to his students. Everybody smiles and waves and smiles again.

The next day's interview is wide ranging. We discuss the Amrit yoga style, yoga competitions and the general direction yoga is headed, before settling in to a discussion of gurus. Desai reminds me that he can't talk about Kripalu, but even when he talks in generalities his answers are intriguing. He tells me that it's a mistake to assume gurus have nothing left to learn. "I may play the role of the guru, perhaps you may respect me as a guru, but I'm always the disciple, the learner, the seeker," he says. "I'm not a finished product. I'm evolving. I'm growing." In other words, gurus are just as liable as regular folks to make mistakes. "In any part of the world anywhere there has never been such a thing as a perfect guru who will never make any mistakes whatsoever," he tells me, before adding something interesting: "And it is not about the guru. It is about who is seeking the perfection as their ultimate protection." Some students unrealistically expect gurus to be perfect, he says, because "they want to have somebody to protect them with that perfection."

Desai's energy starts to flag. He remains cooperative, but I sense his tolerance for my line of questioning is rapidly waning. I ask him about the inherent dangers of the guru-disciple relationship and he dismisses it with a smile. "It depends on you and the teacher. So, it's how you develop your relationship," he says. Another warm smile. The interview is over.

As Yogi Desai heads off to his tiny room I wander back to the main meditation hall with Malay. He insists that "not all of the facts" surrounding the Kripalu case made it out. He doesn't want to elaborate further but reminds me that the events that the charges stem from happened during an "earlier" and "different" time, which I can only presume to mean a time that was more ... *open*?

Where does all this leave the teaching of brahmacharya? Looking through all of the Amrit Yoga Institute's written materials I can't find any mention of this particular yama, except for a recommendation to practice brahmacharya for one week before taking a certain workshop. And I've yet to hear the word mentioned during my time among the Amrit yoga trainees.

As for Kripalu, only new residents are required to practice celibacy and only for a maximum of two years. "In the early days we were so focused on celibacy—we held it as such a central value—that we created a charge around it," Kripalu's board of trustees chair Richard Faulds told *Yoga Journal.* "Brahmacharya was overemphasized, and to the extent that we enforced it as a lifestyle, we created dysfunction. People have a tendency, when they're having such a basic urge denied, to express it in some other, less-than-straightforward, inappropriate ways," he added. "Our experience, looking back, is that celibacy is not a healthy long-term lifestyle for most people."[6] Call me a depraved hedonist, but I could have told you that.

Everybody is immersed in training during my last day at the Zen Center. I watch a little knot of prospective teachers correcting each other's poses. Another clump is sitting in silent meditation. The whole scene has an odd, out-of-time feel; there's the studied discipleship and overt earnestness that I've come to associate with the quintessential sixties yoga experience, yet it also has that streamlined hum that characterizes so much of the modern yoga business. I chat to a few students about their connection to "Gurudev." "Yogi Amrit Desai is the top yogi," a trainee named Nancy tells me. "My mission is to spread his love through myself, and that's what I intend to do." Julie, an Australian yoga teacher who had traveled to the United

States to study with Desai, explains it this way: "It's just happened that I really connect with his teachings *and* I connect with him. I think he's from the heart. He's sincere."

All of the students I speak to are familiar with, yet untroubled by, Yogi Desai's past. "If you ask for people to be perfect, even gurus, then you're setting yourself up for a fall, because nothing's perfect," Julie says. "When he walks off the stage, off the chair, he's a human being. He's got a personality. He's a father. And so he's on the path, just like we all are." She smiles at me and her eyes twinkle. "The whole guru thing gets very misunderstood."

In Gurus We Trust

Nowadays just about anybody in the public eye is a candidate for deification. Consider the feted fleet of financial, fashion and fitness "gurus" who flit across our television screens nightly. This drive to exalt is in the North American DNA, says journalist and yogi Andrew Vontz. "There are many people who follow gurus and cultish leaders in all kinds of strange ways and we treat them as though they're normal.… People revere Bill Gates and George Bush and Rush Limbaugh and do we get upset and think that they're complete freaks?" Vontz asks (although this is hardly the rhetorical slam-dunk it's intended to be).

Nowhere is this culture-wide system of virtually assured veneration more marked than in the American spiritual marketplace, where things are absolutely bonkers. Emboldened by the American Constitution's ironclad prohibition on any regulation of religion, the world's swamis, shamans and soothsayers have long flocked to the United States to mix it up with our best homegrown snake-handlers and self-helpers. And why not? This is where the action is, not to mention the money. Westerners in general have a tendency to jump heart first, while Americans in particular have proven time and again to be the most willing of believers, often displaying a steadfast refusal to separate what is spiritual from what is human.

Of all the imports, India's holy men and women, with their exotic mantras, flowing saffron robes and pantheon of gods, have consistently outperformed their opponents. This explains why there are more ashrams and Zen Centers strewn across North America than, say, Zoroastrian fire temples. And while gurudom's halcyon days may have passed into memory, and many of the most influential leaders have passed on, a number of Indian leaders exert impressive sway over their followers to this day. Even Bikram Choudhury, who rejects the "guru" label and certainly never pretends to be a great spiritual teacher, has a cadre of ardent acolytes. "Ultimately, I still have my free will, always, and there are things that I would not do if Bikram told me to," says Bikramite and yoga champion Esak Garcia. "But for the most part I will do anything that he wants. I trust him. I believe in him."

Yet despite our embrace of South Asian spiritualism, there's something about the teacher-student relationship at the core of many of these beliefs that westerners find difficult to navigate. Diane Featherstone is a certified Kripalu yoga teacher, thirty-year yoga practitioner and cofounder of the Frog Pond Yoga Centre in Massachusetts. Sitting in her living room (earth tones, djembe drum, Native American dreamcatcher on the wall), talking gurus, she says it's not the relationship itself that's the problem but the tunnel vision typical of many westerners. "People aren't taught to think for themselves. Or aren't given the freedom and the liberty to find their own truth as children. You know there are so many ways we indoctrinate people—the family, the schools, the churches, economics, the color of your skin, your nationality, your creed. So people grow up not knowing who they are," she says. "So when people start this practice, they suddenly meet this person [the guru]. And they don't know who it is. Or who they are. And that can be traumatic for them."

"The guru-disciple tradition is not well understood in the West," says Trisha Lamb with typical understatement. Herself a follower of the Buddhist guru Garchen Rinpoche, she says it may have something to do with the independent streak common among westerners. "The guru-disciple relationship is portrayed as parent-child. When it's functioning in its mature form it doesn't work like that," she says. One hundred years of salacious headlines probably aren't doing the relationship any favors either, from the "Omnipotent Oom" we met earlier all the way up to "Sexy Sadie." "They [outsiders] see it as cultish, when it isn't really. It's just because there's not an in-depth enough understanding of how the process works," Lamb contends.

Diane Featherstone studied yoga in India and says witnessing the enormous differences between the two cultures has helped her understand the ruptures that occur so frequently in this relationship, especially regarding sex. "In India, the gurus are so cloistered, and they have these gatherings where the men sit on one side and the women sit on the other side. And the women are, you know, most modestly clothed. And they don't have that right-up-in-your-face interaction with the gurus. And then they [the gurus] come to this country …" Featherstone raises her eyebrows. "It probably is an experience they never had before." Although that's no excuse, she says, for those "bad apple" gurus who use this asymmetrical power dynamic to their advantage. "Those kinds of relationships demand huge respect and trust. And one of the greatest, most painful experiences, according to therapists, is the experience of betrayal. And that's what it is, a betrayal." Featherstone has a great name for this kind of charlatan in swami's robes. "They're called the Phony Holies."

The Phony Holies

From time immemorial we have looked for the deity in human form, someone who can absolve us of responsibility, someone to whom we can abdicate the often-crushing weight of daily decisions and judgments. This law of spiritual supply and demand prevails in the East, where self-proclaimed holy men crowd the landscape. Yet the simple laws of probability tell us that not all of these guys can possibly be the real deal. "There have been God men and gurus in India for hundreds of years, and probably the Indians are more adept at debunking them than anyone," cult intervention expert Rick Ross tells me. "Westerners are more easily taken in than Indians, who are used to these folks."[7]

So who's to blame for the swarm of sham swamis that have washed up on our shores? According to Swami Muktananda, it's the followers' fault. "We choose our Gurus just as we choose our politicians. The false Guru market is growing because the false disciple market is growing," the swami was once quoted as saying. "A true disciple would never be trapped by a false Guru."[8] What about the experiences followers have under a false guru? Are they still valid? Can a person make spiritual progress under a corrupt master? The Bhagwan Shree Rajneesh once claimed it was "better to have perfect faith in an imperfect master than imperfect faith in a perfect master"—although he *would* say that, given how comically imperfect he was (more about him in the next chapter).[9]

Manhattan psychotherapist Dan Shaw considered himself one of Muktananda's true disciples. He met Muktananda in the late seventies, during the swami's third world tour. Just a few years earlier Muktananda had been another obscure spiritualist in the jungle north of Bombay. This swami was developing a new religious movement based on his reading of Siddha yoga, a relatively recent yoga lineage focused on meditation, chanting, volunteer service and offerings to the guru. Around this time Americans such as former-Harvard-professor-turned-spiritual-teacher Ram Dass and former-car-salesman-turned-Human Potential-leader Werner Erhard were roaming the Indian countryside in search of gurus. Dass and Erhard became enamored of Muktananda. A marriage was made in heaven, and Dass and Erhard decided to sponsor Muktananda on a tour of North America.

America suited Muktananda and vice versa. By the mid-seventies he'd already established a western headquarters for Siddha yoga, converting an old resort hotel two hours north of New York City in a has-been corner of the Catskill Mountains known as the Borscht Belt into a sprawling ashram—the same ashram I mentioned at the beginning of this chapter that I tried to visit. Muktananda also set up a nonprofit foundation called Siddha Yoga Dham of America (SYDA), charged with propagating Muktananda's teachings and running other Siddha yoga ashrams.

SYDA's upstate ashram was mushrooming, bringing other groups and other gurus with it. "By the eighties they had three hotels on contiguous properties, busloads and planeloads of people. It was quite a scene," recalls Dan Shaw. SYDA was also making great inroads into the worlds of art, entertainment and politics. *Time* magazine reported that by 1976 SYDA had attracted over twenty thousand devotees, including banner names such as John Denver, Phylicia Rashad, James Taylor, Carly Simon and former California governor Jerry Brown.[10] The Borscht Belt had been transformed into what *The New York Times* now calls the Bhajan Belt, an area of loosely affiliated holistic businesses, yoga retreats and back-to-nature enterprises.[11] Muktananda's main Indian ashram also thrived in the reflected heat of its radiant Western counterparts. "They brought a lot of Western glamour to that little tiny village in India," Shaw says.

Shaktipat was and remains the spiritual ace up SYDA's sleeve. A rite honored in many religious and yogic traditions, shaktipat is the transmission of spiritual power from guru to disciple, aimed at awakening the cosmic energy known as shakti, which supposedly resides at the base of the spine. At SYDA ashrams these transmissions occur during shaktipat "intensives," annual one-day events that cost around $500. Lucky beneficiaries described Muktananda's shaktipats as a blissful, even ecstatic experience. "In the climactic moment, the guru places his fingers on the disciple's closed eyes and gently pushes the head back and forth. The disciple is then supposed to feel the power flowing into him as if by an electric charge. Some people say they have experienced flashing lights, visions, ethereal sounds, and even, among women, orgasm," *Time* magazine reported.[12]

One wonders what the husbands and lovers who couldn't make it to Shakti Day thought of the whole orgasm angle. They certainly wouldn't have been too impressed if they'd been privy to all the facts, which, of course, came out only later. For, it turns out, shaktipat wasn't the only transmission going on at Muktananda's ashrams.

To the outside world, Swami Muktananda was recognized as a great *Brahmachari* who had long ago taken a vow of celibacy and asceticism, in line with the teachings of traditional Siddha yoga. Muktananda believed in brahmacharya so much that he even asked his supporters to follow suit, telling a gathering at the New York ashram in 1972, "What you need is this strength, this seminal vigor. Therefore I insist on total celibacy as long as you are staying in the ashram."[13] But what was good for the guru was not always good for the groupie, it seems.

Muktananda died of a heart attack in October 1982 at age seventy-four. The timing might have been fortuitous. Just a few months later a devastating article in the winter 1983 edition of

CoEvolution Quarterly (later renamed *Whole Earth Review*) blew the lid off life inside SYDA and forever stained Muktananda's legacy. In the article, titled "The Secret Life of Swami Muktananda," writer William Rodarmor asserts that Muktananda regularly had sex with underaged female devotees, claims backed up by months of research and interviews with twenty-five present and former devotees. These charge made the other accusations leveled at Muktananda in the article (ferocious temper, physically abusive, miserly with money, obsessed with celebrity, slept with a shotgun, employed "enforcers") seem like schoolboy taunts. Worse yet, the guru's sexual exploits were common knowledge around the ashram, one ex-devotee told Rodarmor. "It was supposed to be Muktananda's big secret … but since many of the girls were in their early to middle teens, it was hard to keep it secret," the ex-devotee said.[14]

The article profiled a victim of Muktananda's identified only as "Jennifer" who alleged that Muktananda raped her at SYDA's main Indian ashram in 1978. Jennifer claims that Muktananda ordered her to his room late at night, told her to disrobe and had intercourse with her for an hour. "He kept saying, 'Sixty minutes,'" she is quoted as saying in the article. "He claimed he was using the real Indian positions, not the Westernized ones used in America." A devastated Jennifer made plans to escape the ashram even as Muktananda continued to hound her. "He used to watch me getting undressed through the keyhole," she told Rodarmor.

The article also recounted the story of "Mary," who claimed that she was seduced by Muktananda at the New York ashram when she was in her early twenties. (He was seventy-three.) "He didn't have an erection," Rodarmor quoted Mary as saying, "but he inserted about as much as he could. He was standing up, and his eyes were rolled up to the ceiling. He looked as if he was in some sort of ecstasy." Mary was ordered back to the guru's room the next day and suffered through the same ordeal. She also claimed that Muktananda had a secret passageway from his house to the young girls' dormitory and alleged that at least eight other young girls told her they'd had sex with him. "I knew that he had girls marching in and out of his bedroom all night long," she said. Mary later confided in one of Muktananda's long-time translators, a young and beautiful woman named Malti Shetty. According to Mary, Malti didn't seem surprised, and said that "people had been coming to her with this for years and years" and she was "caught in the middle."

It was a disturbing pattern, to say the least. Charges would be aired against Muktananda and his followers would find a way to rationalize or diminish his poor behavior. Some adherents even claimed Muktananda's actions were justified because he wasn't ejaculating into the girls, an abhorrent line of logic that had something to do with "conserving Kundalini energy." SYDA devotees even managed to turn their heads when an SYDA swami, quitting the ashram in disgust, put his reasons on paper in an open letter. "I believe that when a Guru begins to lose sight of moral values—whether because of senility, madness, illness, or whatever reason—and regards others as objects to manipulate and use for his own ends … it is a disciple's DUTY to leave that Guru," the Swami wrote. "It is therefore with much regret and deep anguish that I feel forced to terminate my discipleship to you. May God protect and guide you."[15]

Around this time, just two hours away from the ashram in bustling New York, Dan Shaw was busy being intensely unhappy. "I was desperately looking for some kind of direction or hope," he says. (He was an actor at the time. I could have told him, from experience, what a miserable lot that can be.) Shaw began making regular trips to the ashram, and remembers being dazzled by the effect Muktananda had on his followers: "It was a big crowd, kind of like at a rock concert, chanting in awe. It was exciting and alluring and I started to feel happier and more purposeful."

Muktananda's version of Siddha yoga was intensely guru-centric. "There is no deity superior to the guru, no gain better than the guru's grace … no state higher than meditation on the guru," Rodarmor quoted Muktananda as saying. *Siddha guru* literally means "perfect master," and Muktananda made sure everyone know just how perfect he was, says Dan Shaw. "Muktananda made it quite clear that he was God and was to be treated as such. He could therefore do anything he wanted to do.… If it was cruel, if it was exploitative, if it was illegal, if it was destructive, it was God's will."

But God was getting on. By the early eighties it was time to pass the torch. Muktananda eventually chose as his successor none other than Malti Shetty, the young woman to whom Muktananda's alleged victim Mary had brought her accusations. Malti, then aged twenty-six, was renamed Chidvilasananda ("bliss of the play of consciousness"), took the vows of monkhood and set off down the boulevard of brahmacharya. Today devotees call her by the honorific Gurumayi, meaning "one who is absorbed in the guru." She is revered as a majestic and mystical leader, head of SYDA's vast spiritual empire, boasting more than 550 meditation centers worldwide. And Gurumayi is not your average wizened swami. Descriptions of her (beyond the requisite "warm," "humorous" and "joyful") are almost always along the lines of "startlingly glamorous" or "radiantly beautiful," as if reference to her corporeal beauty is required. Meanwhile, her dwindling public appearances and reticence to talk to people like me have only added to the air of mystery and inscrutability that surrounds her, like a Hindu Howard Hughes.

During Gurumayi's reign, SYDA would continue to be roiled by controversies, mostly carnal (still?) and mostly involving a Lebanese-born devotee and close confidant of Gurumayi's named George Afif. In California in 1983 Afif was charged with burglary and statutory rape of a teenage girl, the daughter of prominent SYDA followers. Afif, who was married at the time to a woman who lived at the New York ashram, pleaded no contest to the statutory rape charge and was sentenced to a suspended six-month jail term and three years' probation. However, the conviction was expunged after Afif served probation according to California law. A few years later Afif spearheaded the attempt to rebuild a small lake at the New York ashram. In an open letter posted on an anti-SYDA website, ex-devotees claim the effort "has proven to be a fiscal and public relations fiasco," with SYDA being forced to pay enormous fines for environmental damage the project has caused.[16] (Verifying these claims has proven difficult. And at least they don't involve teenage girls.)

Despite never holding any official position with SYDA, Afif seemed to exert extraordinary influence over events within the organization. "It was hard to tell who was running things. Was it George? Was it Gurumayi?" Shaw says. Many ex-members claim Afif derived his power from a romantic, possibly even sexual, relationship with Gurumayi.[17] This would, of course, be a flagrant violation of Gurumayi's vow of brahmacharya, although none of the claims has ever been substantiated. What *is* known is that Afif vanished from the SYDA scene around 1994, soon after Lakegate. Afif is no longer affiliated with SYDA and my efforts to reach him have not been successful.

The good news, according to Dan Shaw, is that the well-documented sexual and financial scrapes that happened on Muktananda's watch largely subsided over time. The bad news is that they were replaced by equally egregious abuses, this time overseen by Gurumayi. Shaw claims that ashram leaders routinely abused privacy and confidentiality to their advantage. "Gurumayi often publicly humiliated people by revealing things that they found embarrassing," Shaw says. Other abuses ran to the exotic. Shaw claims smuggling was common between the Indian and American ashrams: "There was a lot of travel back and forth, and people were given all kinds of jewelry or cash to hide on their body or in their luggage." And, Shaw says, followers were too busy pleasing the guru to ask questions or consider the repercussions. "I once arrived in the middle of the night in the Bombay airport with four giant trunks full of stuff, and I had no idea what was in it, and I had to explain myself to customs," he recalls. The surprise cargo turned out to be benign (castor oil, one of the various unguents Gurumayi supposedly required to sate various evolving health fetishes). But it could have been worse, as Shaw later discovered. "There was a huge bag full of money, which they never found. I was lucky for that," he says.

The most serious abuse Shaw witnessed, and one that he says continues today inside SYDA and similar organizations, is the psychological abuse that leaders inflict on followers. "There's a vast amount of underlying cruelty: the wish to control, enslave and keep them [followers] under control through shame and fear," Shaw says. "It's packaged and sold as the way to enlightenment. So the voluntary enslavement of the desires of the group becomes a way to enlightenment. People are not brainwashed or hypnotized into this, but they are seduced."

It wouldn't be the first time.

Cult Following

Mention the word *cult* and inflammatory images fill your head; Jonestown, Charles Manson, Waco. Mention yoga and people think incense. But your average yoga group has more in common with a cult than many yogis would like to believe, says cult intervention specialist Rick Ross. Ross began tracking cult activity in 1982, after a group targeting Jews for conversion to Pentecostalism infiltrated his grandmother's nursing home. His focus is destructive cults, groups that share three main characteristics: an authoritarian leader with no meaningful accountability, followers who have handed over the process of thinking for themselves to this leader, and the harming of others, anything from financial exploitation to physical or even sexual abuse. And according to Ross, some of these groups have "hitched a ride on the yoga craze. They're seeing yoga as a means of recruitment." In these groups, Ross explains, the focus is often on the guru to the point that it becomes "all about the leader, as opposed to spirituality or yoga or some other practice."

Nobody is suggesting that mass-suicide nuts have colonized the entire yoga industry or that the business has become one enormous cover for occult worship. Even Ross is quick to point out that it's just a small sliver of the industry. But this tiny minority has the potential to do great harm, says Dan Shaw. "Within the yoga universe some people are wrestling with the idea of purification. 'Can I purify my mind, my heart, my body, my breath?' Whenever you start to aspire to that kind of perfection of purification you enter that danger zone where you can become obsessive. You can start dichotomizing good and evil," he says. "When that idea arises, certain groups of people have to be despised; it can be rationalized that they have to be killed and destroyed."

Ross says people just need to be careful that they're not biting off more than they can metaphysically chew. "Most of the people that are interested in yoga in Western industrial countries see it as a form of exercise. I question that what they really want to do is reshape their spirituality or their conscious mind or their subconscious mind. So what they need to do is examine that group that they are signing up for," he says. "Many times people are just plain tricked.

There's a kind of bait-and-switch process where what people think they're joining is not really what they get into."

It's also easy to assume, says Shaw, that only weak-willed nobodies are attracted to groups such as SYDA, which he calls a "soft-core cult." In fact, the opposite is more often the case. "The average participant is a quite accomplished, college-educated, middle-class person. There were many very wealthy people there, heirs and heiresses. There were many descendants of the founding fathers of this country who were living full time in the ashram," Shaw says. Rick Ross adds, "I've been dealing with cult victims for over twenty years, and I've never been able to distinguish a single personality profile"—except that they are usually highly educated, young and healthy. "People who can be productive, so they can be useful to a group," he says.

The more important question is *how* all these savorers of culture, these dedicated readers of *The Nation*, these supporters of free inquiry and democracy could find themselves so deeply enmeshed in destructive organizations? For the famous, the influential and the powerful, it makes some sort of sense. "Celebrities are, for a cult group, instant cachet and recognition," Ross says. Because this helps recruit new converts, cult groups often work very hard to lure big names with the red-carpet treatment. Shaw says that SYDA had a very specific outreach aimed at securing famous followers: "We would contact celebrities, VIPs and influential people and invite them to special gatherings to talk to them about Gurumayi."

For Everyday Joes the process of indoctrination is usually gradual. Rick Ross likens it to a frog being boiled in a pot of water, not realizing until too late that it should leap out. Shaw remembers joining SYDA when he was vulnerable and desperate for relief. "Relief from despair, from psychological despair, depression, frustration, hopelessness, emptiness.... I was having a rough time and I was not finding much relief from anything," he says. In contrast, ashram life was intoxicating and offered instant community. A few personal disappointments later and his fate was sealed. "I said, 'That's it! Why don't I become a religious person? Maybe I'll be become a monk,

Shop Till You Drop

You can capture a little SYDA magic for yourself by visiting the organization's store. But don't forget your wallet.

DVDs
Wherever You Are Attain the Self, $24.95
Trust—The Siddha Yoga message for 2003 by Gurumayi, $39.95

Photography and Art
16 x 20-inch photograph of Muktananda, $125
6 x 8-foot reproduction of the painting *Trust Is Transcendent*, mounted on acid-free white mat board, $2,700

Jewelry/Clothing
Sandalwood neck mala, $125
Pearl neck mala, $795
Aquamarine wrist mala, $495
Gurumayi signature ring, gold, $299
Jacquard shawl, pashmina cashmere, $149

maybe I'll become a missionary' … So I packed up and said a 'goodbye cruel world' kind of thing."

And in some cases, it's simple yoga that gets potential devotees through the front door. Ross cites the story of Catherine Cheng. In 1998 twenty-three-year-old Cheng had a fiancé, a loving family and, as a promising law student in New York, an excellent career ahead of her. "I want to become a great, effective, litigating lawyer and strive for justice," Cheng wrote at the time. She was also practicing yoga at a Manhattan studio run by the Integral Yoga Institute, the group founded by so-called Woodstock guru Swami Satchidananda. In December 1998 Cheng began a month-long yoga retreat at the institute's main Yogaville ashram in rural Virginia. Her boyfriend told her to be careful; he'd heard about some yoga groups that were accused of being cults. "If these people are weird, I'll leave. I'm too smart to get caught up in that," she told him.[18]

Catherine Cheng never returned. "In a matter of weeks she cut off meaningful communication with family and friends," Ross recounts. Even more troubling, she broke off her relationship with her boyfriend and announced she was marrying a man named Larry Gross, a swami at the ashram who she'd known for just two weeks. Gross, who also happened to be one of Yogaville's lawyers, told peers he planned to give up his vows of brahmacharya to marry Cheng.

The Cheng family was eventually able to arrange one meeting at Yogaville with their daughter, with Rick Ross present. The meeting did not go well. "Catherine Cheng, in my opinion, had been subjected to the group for so long and so intensely that she just wasn't critically thinking or interacting with her family in a meaningful way anymore. She would sit in almost a trance-like state for hours, barely communicating," Ross says. His latest information is that Catherine Cheng is still active with Yogaville and may have a child, although it's believed she may be separated from her swami husband. She remains estranged from her family. "It was one of the most radical cases I've ever dealt with in my career," Ross says. "And it all started by nothing more than by taking yoga classes in Manhattan."

SYDA continues to make news. In 2007 it joined forces with a local homeowners group in a lawsuit to stop a large-scale building project in the small town of Fallsburg, where the SYDA ashram is located. In its suit, SYDA alleges the town had (wait for it) "failed to conduct proper environmental reviews for such a large-scale project." According to the article, local legislators were up in arms that SYDA, a nonprofit religious organization that's exempt from paying property taxes, had challenged the project.[19] And in 2002 SYDA announced up to 250 job cuts after rumors began swirling that the ashram was looking to leave upstate New York for California. A SYDA spokesman announced it would stay put, but only after the foundation was "reconfigured to better serve the community."[20] SYDA was even linked with Hollywood star Meg Ryan, if you can believe the *National Enquirer*. According to the *Enquirer*, Ryan and former husband Dennis Quaid had squabbled during their 2001 divorce over who would get to "keep" Gurumayi. Ryan was a devotee first and thought it was only proper that her estranged husband move on to a different swami. (One wonders if it was the buffed, nipped and tucked Ms. Ryan who introduced Gurumayi to the wonders of plastic surgery, which ex-devotees claim she has undergone.)[21]

It's not all bad news. SYDA's profile and credibility are boosted by the involvement of John Friend, the influential and well-regarded founder of the increasingly popular Anusara yoga style, who considers Gurumayi his guru.[22] And despite mountains of negative press, the SYDA ashram continues to attract a wide swath of believers from all walks of life, including the young, educated professionals and artists from Manhattan who have always formed its core. (I know of one urbane New Yorker who keeps a small shrine to Gurumayi in her bedroom.) Gurumayi does manage to have a public profile, despite making almost no personal appearances. She figures most notably, albeit anonymously, in the pages of Elizabeth Gilbert's bestselling book *Eat, Pray, Love*. Gilbert describes seeing "a photograph of this stunning Indian woman" who would become her guru and, later, going to live at an ashram where followers "pay tribute to a statue of a Siddha Yogi (or "perfected master") who established this lineage."[23]

It's obvious that I'm not going to get an interview with Gurumayi or anyone else at SYDA. That's okay. I won't be the last writer looking to get inside her head. Even with SYDA's worst days behind it, in the internet age the organization can never escape its past, with each new flare-up threatening to reignite previous scandals. I even begin to feel a little sorry for SYDA as I consider the number of writers, bloggers and ex-devotees piling on the organization. People such as Dan Shaw, who are just waiting for the curtain to drop. "It seems inevitable that if you set yourself up to be an omnipotent deity, it is likely to be shown at some point that the emperor has no clothes," he says with a grin.

With a little time up my sleeve, I decide to dig a little farther through some of these web pages, many of which I've visited countless times. The farther I dig, the more an unsettling trend reveals itself: Followers have a guru relationship go sour, find the strength to get out but then turn around and go right back into a similar guru relationship. Like the battered woman who won't leave her abuser, these former devotees recount in excruciating detail their brave escape from the clutches of a false prophet, only to end their gripping narratives with the deflating news that they've found a new guru. (The story of Shannon Jo Ryan, the daughter of U.S. Representative Leo Ryan, who was slain in 1978 while investigating the Jonestown cult in Guyana, unfolded along similarly sad lines. Ryan was raised Catholic but by her early twenties had rejected the Church and was instead, she said, "getting into holistic health and looking for something that had meaning." In 1980, after studying transpersonal counseling in California, Ryan visited the spiritual leader Bhagwan Shree Rajneesh at his short-lived Montclair, New Jersey, ashram. In 1981, just three years after her father's death at the hands of a cult, she announced she had become the Bhagwan's disciple.[24] Shannon's sister Patricia, meanwhile, went on to become president of the Cult Awareness Network.)

For the Beatles, who provided many westerners with their first exposure to the ancient ideas of the East when they became followers of the Maharishi Mahesh Yogi in 1968, one guru was enough. Once they'd decided the Maharishi was not all he was cracked up to be, the Fab Four never went back. Harrison remained a dabbler in Eastern mysticism until his death, but never again with the Maharishi, while John Lennon became a hero to heretics, atheists and agnostics worldwide by writing anthemic lyrics that asked us to imagine a world with no heaven.

It's ironic that the Beatles were given so much blame/credit for propagating Eastern religion, yoga and the whole free-love ethos, when in fact they'd mostly disassociated themselves from it. (George Harrison, the most spiritually inclined of the four, once described San Francisco's hippies as "hideous, spotty little teenagers.")[25] And in the irony-on-irony department, Rick Ross reminds me that the Maharishi's career—and wallet—continued to blossom even *after* his horrible public breakup with the Beatles. "Maharishi didn't just fade away like a fool on the hill. He went on to become a bigger guru than ever and to have followers all over the world," Ross says. He claims the late Maharishi's empire is estimated at between $5 and $9 billion, while the combined Beatles' estate is estimated at less than $2 billion. Who's laughing now?

Tap That Asana

Another scandal recently rocked yoga. This wasn't some minor indignity relegated to the opinion column of *Yoga Journal* or part of an obscure thesis paper. This was an uproar that played out across the front pages. This controversy didn't have the stale whiff of counterculture days gone by. It was a thoroughly modern tumult, much better suited to the here and now. Most important, this affront didn't involve some grizzled old grandpa in a kaftan, no sir. This outrage engulfed none other than the stud-muffin of yoga.

Rodney Yee is American yoga royalty, the handsome, long-haired, lighthearted poster boy for everything the mainstream loves about yoga. His instructional DVDs outsell Hollywood blockbusters, his appearance on magazine covers virtually guarantees a spike in sales and his in-person classes are full of twitchy female fans clamoring for an "adjustment." Yee is teaching a series of classes at the Omega Institute for Holistic Studies in upstate New York, one of America's most prominent New Age institutions. We've decided I'll drive there to meet him, to discuss his career ups and downs.

It's been mostly ups. At age fifty-one, Yee has been at the yoga game a comparatively long time. The youngest of five children born to an air force colonel father and homemaker mother, Yee was a typical army brat growing up, moving between military bases in California, Oklahoma and Puerto Rico. Yee was a gymnast and committed ballet dancer, even giving up his philosophy major once in college to pursue ballet full time. He began studying Iyengar yoga in 1981 and was teaching at a studio called the Yoga Room in Berkeley just a few years later. "I started yoga when it wasn't really popular. I had many years where I was a waiter and a yoga teacher. I was a dancer and a yoga teacher. I was a lot of different things at the same time," he says. "You'd be in the South and you'd say, 'I'm a yoga teacher,' and they'd say 'Yogurt? What?'" Around this time Yee started dating a fellow yogi by the name of Donna Fone. (Typical date: yoga class and dinner.) Yee was determined to make a living from his new passion and in 1987 cofounded the Piedmont Yoga Studio in California, which he ran with Fone, now his wife and later to become mother of his three children. The studio was (and remains) a success, and Yee's reputation spread.

The nineties belonged to Yee. He became the most recognizable face in the industry, starring in a series of big-selling instructional DVDs that traded on his good looks and easy charm. With Fone he released another set of DVDs with feel-good titles such as *Yoga for Two* and *Family Yoga*. In January 2001 *Yoga Journal* profiled Yee and Fone for the magazine's "Yoga Couples" series, declaring that they'd "found yoga to be the foundation of their marriage." "It's a balancing act," Fone told the magazine, "with Rodney at the prime of his career, me at the helm of the business, and both of us at the heart of the family."[26]

Yee's appeal was about to cross over. An April 2001 appearance on Oprah Winfrey's eponymous talk show catapulted Yee into the mainstream. (What *hasn't* Oprah catapulted into the mainstream?) "It sent things into a whole different orbit," Yee says. "It blew everything off the map." Including Russell Crowe. Days after the *Oprah* appearance, one of Yee's titles replaced *Gladiator* as Amazon.com's top-selling DVD. Stories began cropping up in mainstream newspapers and magazines about his celebrity clientele, including Demi Moore and Mariel Hemingway. "I've introduced Rodney to many of my friends," clothing designer Donna Karan told *People* magazine. "Everyone falls in love with him. It's this big crush."[27] *Time* magazine even christened him the "studmuffin guru," a label that's stuck despite Yee's protestations.[28] It's not the studmuffin part he objects to. "What man in this world doesn't want to be called a studmuffin?" he asks. It's the label "guru" that bothers him. "Then you're upping the ante," he says.

You see, Rodney Yee never wanted to be in the guru business. His entirely contemporary brand of yoga is aimed at enhancing your life without messing up your *lifestyle*; you can still drive a car, you can hold down a regular job, you don't have to live in a mountaintop retreat. For those who embrace this interpretation of yoga, the job of guru is little more than a relic of the past, much like radio DJs. "I don't think 'the guru' or gurus are totally necessary," Yee tells me. "Initially it feels good. It's a stroke to the ego, to have people bow to you. [But] to me, it's just isolating. It puts you up on a pedestal."

And we all know what happens to gurus who sit high atop pedestals.

"Yoga Guru in Compromising Position" screamed the headline of a front-page story in the May 12, 2002, *San Francisco Chronicle*. The article claimed that a former instructor at Yee's Piedmont studio had filed a breach-of-contract lawsuit against Yee and the studio, alleging that Yee and his wife had terminated the instructor's lease after she had accused Yee of having affairs with female students. The accusations of affairs were corroborated by two of Yee's former students, who both said they'd had a sexual relationship with Yee that lasted several months. "Rodney's misrepresentations to me, to other students and to his family about his sexual involvement with students represents an abuse of power and is unbecoming of a healer or a teacher," one of the women declared. "His refusal to accept that he needs help in this area and his attempts to blame the women involved puts more students at risk." For his part, Yee claimed the case was retaliation for "firing someone who was basically bad-mouthing me." Yee says he offered the former instructor the opportunity to meet with a third party to resolve the dispute and says it was only after she declined the offer that he asked her to leave the studio.[29]

Yee later admitted to extramarital meanderings in the April 2004 issue of *SELF* magazine (an unlikely recipient for this sort of scoop, if ever there was one). All writers and filmmakers appreciate subjects who tackle questions head-on, but even I'd be hard-pressed to say Yee did himself any favors in this interview. "The reality is that most teachers fall in love with their students, but sex is such a small part of it," Yee told the magazine. "I've never had one-night affairs, but deep friendships that moved into sexuality. If that's a mistake, then I've made that mistake," he continued. There was more. "But what about when two consenting adults decide to get into something and there's no coercion? Until we change the law, I don't understand what the big deal is. It's private. It's none of your business or anyone else's." Yee even tried to turn conventional wisdom on its head, suggesting that the perceived power imbalance between a female student and male teacher favors the student. "Who owns the key to the door?" he asked. "A woman—she decides."[30]

The case eventually settled out of court "to the satisfaction of all parties," according to a spokeswoman for Yee.[31] (The terms of the settlement are sealed.) However, as usual with these situations, the facts of the case were irrelevant. It was all about *whom.* There'd been plenty of yoga scandals before, but never involving someone with Yee's high public profile. The Golden Boy was about to be taken down a notch. His career was over. At least that's how the script went.

In real life it unfolded a little differently. Times have changed. The kind of scandal that was guaranteed to have caused an uproar in the past had become old news. In today's increasingly sexualized yoga business, it's simply no big deal that yoga teachers act like rock stars. Why not? We've given them license to. Sure, the yoga discussion boards did register a requisite amount of outrage. Some indignant old-time yogis hooted and hollered about the latest battering brahmacharya had taken. Calls for the yoga industry to adopt an enforceable code of ethics were trotted out once again. But by and large the hullabaloo just sort of blew over. The case resolved, Yee threw out some quotable quotes and life went on. "Sometimes the guru relationship gets in the way. I make mistakes, you make mistakes. Hopefully, we get back up, we learn from them. And we move on," Yee tells me. "I took my tumbles and falls, and I'm where I stand now because of it."

Having walked away from that ruckus relatively clean, Yee perhaps suddenly felt bulletproof. The fuss from the *SELF* magazine article had only just died down when there was Yee, canoodling all over the pages of *New York* magazine with his new girlfriend, model and yoga instructor Colleen Saidman, discussing how they'd hooked up despite the fact that both were still married. (Someone get these guys a new press agent!) They *did* seem to be a pretty good match. She's a bendy hottie with her own studio in the Hamptons, the New York elite's summer getaway of choice, and a roster of celeb clients— Christie Brinkley! Russell Simmons! He's Rodney Yee. She left her husband of twenty-four years to be with him. He left his wife of twenty-four years to be with her. Perfect on paper.

Saidman was gracious enough to point out that her relationship with Yee should not be an example to anyone else in the yoga world, warning that teachers "shouldn't go there. Even though we did." And she admitted that the whole thing grossed out more than a few of her students. "I've had people who won't speak to me anymore," she confessed. "It's like I destroyed them. One woman left town." At this point the ick! reflex gave way to the huh? reflex, as the banter careered off into what must be, for these two, the perilous conversational terrain of fidelity. "I trust him at this point," Saidman said. "Maybe that's ridiculous, but I have to." "We both have to," Yee retorted. "And yet we both don't." Yee then assured us that he was no longer prone to temptation "partly because I'm satisfied." "Because I'd kill him otherwise," Saidman replied. "No," Yee continued, "because I'm satisfied."[32] And on and on.

The next time I see Yee and Saidman it's in person, at an Omega yoga conference in New York. He's dressed in blue denims and looking typically studly. She seems (somehow) taller, thinner and blonder than I expected. They've got their hands all over each other. It's sickly but probably smart.

The pair next showed up in *The New York Times,* in a splashy January 2007 story about their wedding day. The article managed to be both rhapsodic and spicy, describing how "the bride glowed more and more throughout the ceremony, as if on a dimmer switch" while also detailing how this platonic relationship suddenly kicked into nonplatonic high gear in a hot tub after a yoga conference.[33] I'll spare you the details, but it had something to do with thumbs, foreheads and third eyes.

Yee and Saidman now live together in the Hamptons with their four children, three by Yee's previous marriage and Saidman's daughter. They teach at Yoga Shanti, the popular studio Saidman founded, while Yee continues to pursue his lucrative DVD career. In 2008 the pair also debuted an online yoga club. If you're interested, they often teach together, in person, at places such as the Omega Institute, where Yee and I first met. Their next Omega weekend intensive offers an "exquisite blend of a masculine and a feminine interpretation of yoga." Just don't go there expecting to learn anything about brahmacharya.

11

Broken Om

Renunciation is the very basis upon which ethics
stands.
—SWAMI VIVEKANANDA, *THE COMPLETE WORKS
OF SWAMI VIVEKANANDA*

For Americans, they were dark days. But for spiritualist Deepak Chopra, the aftermath of September 11 was an opportunity. In an email message from Chopra to twenty-two thousand of his fans and picked up on by *The New York Times*, Chopra wrote that it was natural for Americans to be asking questions about religion and the afterlife. "But by the second paragraph," the *Times* noted, "what began as a communiqué of spiritual affinity turned into marketing, plain and simple." Chopra was concerned that the greatest loss of human life on American soil threatened to bury news of his new novel "about love that survives death and suffering," as he described it. "In the hopes that it won't be overlooked in these difficult days, I'd like to bring this story to your attention," Chopra wrote, directing readers to a link where for just $23.95 they could purchase the book. Contacted by the *Times* for comment, Chopra reread the letter—and conceded that its tone was improper. "In hindsight, that letter was totally inappropriate.... It should not have been sent, and I am sorry," he told the *Times*.

Terrorism seemed to present SYDA's spiritual leader, Gurumayi, with an opportunity as well. In the days immediately following the attacks, visitors to the SYDA website could find "suggestions for spiritual support" that included a $108 prayer shawl and either a Gurumayi mantra or lecture on CD *for just $18.95 each*![1] Far be it for me to doubt Gurumayi's good intentions, but if this isn't a stellar example of something very wrong with much of the yoga business, I don't know what is. When is enough enough?

Thou Shalt Not Be Greedy

Aparigraha is yoga's final yama, the last ethical dictate that Patanjali urges us to adhere to. At the superficial level, aparigraha is the antithesis of *parigraha,* the Sanskrit word for "hoarding." This is usually translated as an abstention from possessiveness, greed, selfishness and acquisitiveness. In practice, it might mean eating only food that has been acquired justly and consuming only what's essential for healthy survival. It could mean getting by with fewer clothes, and even then only what polite society dictates, without regard to the whims of fashion. It could mean going without a car and walking to work. It could mean acquiring wealth concomitant with your lifestyle but nothing more. At the deeper mental level, aparigraha is supposed to be a restraint on covetousness, our hunger for power, for status, for bliss. You can see how this might be more difficult.

Renunciation, the act that underpins aparigraha, has a long and distinguished history in India, its influence felt from the political to the spiritual realm and everywhere in between. It has expressed itself in many forms, from the mundane to the momentous. The most durable example of renunciation in Indian history may be the one set by Siddhartha Gautama, whom followers call the Buddha. Born a prince, Siddhartha was destined to a luxurious life. But at age twenty-nine, in what's called "The Great Renunciation," Siddhartha began living as an ascetic. Later he discovered a path of moderation, the "middle way" that led him to eventual enlightenment. Around the turn of the twentieth century the renowned Indian scientist J.C. Bose offered a modern version of renunciation, refusing to patent his most important discoveries on the grounds that the knowledge should be free for all to use and profit from.[2] (His discoveries include a remote wireless signaling device that Italy's Marconi would "invent" just two years later.) For much of the twentieth century Mahatma Gandhi was seen as a living embodiment of renunciation, shedding the trappings of his high station to cut his own hair, do his own laundry and clean the latrines at his ashram. Gandhi called his dispossession "the richest treasure I own. Hence it is perhaps right to say that though I preach poverty, I am a rich man!"[3] And Indians hailed Sonia Gandhi, the widow of slain former Indian prime minister Rajiv Gandhi, when she won the 2004 Indian election for prime minister but refused to accept the position. "It allows her to assume the high moral ground and signal that she was by no means enamoured of power for its own sake," the *Indian Express* asserted. "Indians love and respect no-one more than a renunciate," declared *The Times of India*.[4]

The notion of renunciation has taken root everywhere. Buddhists know it as the theory of nonattachment, the idea that possessions are an obstacle to liberation. It's echoed in the Bible, particularly in Matthew 19:24, where it's noted that it is "easier for a camel to pass through the eye of a needle than for a rich man to enter the kingdom of God." It's rooted in many of those well-worn everyday axioms— "Live simply so that others may simply live" and the like. The idea has particular and growing import among the eco-savvy, who prefer to interpret aparigraha as the minimal use of resources, and thus as environmentally sound doctrine. Aparigraha is also seen as an antidote to the terribly uneven worldwide distribution of wealth. The essential message is so cut and dried—the power of renunciation will diminish and eventually defeat greed—that it's no wonder it's so popular to embrace.

Present-day yogis are particularly inclined to drape themselves in the robes of renunciation. At the drop of a hat they'll offer holier-than-thou homilies about how to live with little. But saying you live by aparigraha is very different from actually living by aparigraha. A strict Jain monk who practices aparigraha, for instance, lives entirely naked with virtually no possessions at all, seeking only the food and shelter required to stay alive. Can't see that happening in Lower Manhattan (although more likely there than anywhere else in the West). Those who take the vow of aparigraha are not supposed to hoard their time and talent. But aside from the odd promotional event, how many free yoga classes do you know about?

Don't get me wrong. I'm not saying this is an easy edict to live by. We live in a consumerocracy, after all, a culture of inane and insatiable desires, fueled by an idiosyncratic strand of loud, unrelenting and highly effective capitalism. It's hard to see where leaving things behind fits in. I'm not even suggesting that aparigraha is a preferable decree to live by. Just as I don't support shutting down our sexual desires to live by brahmacharya, I see no reason to throw out my big-screen TV on a similar gamble aimed at streamlining my spirituality. The argument is merely that it's duplicitous for urban Western yogis to pretend, in their orbits of plenty, that they're really doing with less. Look around the world. Further, it's a mistake to believe that by merely "practicing" yoga you've somehow shaken off the karmic coil of greed. Aparigraha, perhaps more than any other yama, requires work.

Of course, the people who should put renunciation most respectfully on display are often the worst offenders: millionaire prophets who hide inside sumptuous megachurches, yoga gurus who sit atop empires built not on ethics but on chutzpah and CEOs running tax-free "Zen Centers" while earning more than the American president. The central issue here is *balance*. What are those people charged with passing on sacred teachings about asceticism supposed to do with all the worldly goods they acquire from their instruction? It's a question Deepak Chopra himself tackled in a May 2008 column for *The Washington Post* titled "The Amorality of the Free Market." "Greed is a moral bad but a functional good," Chopra noted, detailing how it was "greedy" junk bond investors who got companies such as FedEx and MCI off the ground. "But most of us are caught up in confusion," Chopra continues, "we feel conflicted about what worldly pleasure—and the money that buys gratification of all kinds—might be doing to our souls."[5] And if we as hosts aren't able to rein in our greed, why should we expect it of our guests, the gurus?

Lost in Translation

It's stunning, the sheer number of Holy Rollers in modern-day America who've given in to their lust for power, money and control.

But even among this colorful competition, Bhagwan Shree Rajneesh and his band of giddy miscreants stand out. The Rajneeshees, as they became known, were the central players in a strange saga of greed, hypocrisy and hubris, a story of aparigraha gone horribly wrong—and a sadly fitting denouement to our journey through the business of yoga.

He was the best of gurus, he was the worst of gurus. Known later in life as Osho and intermittently calling himself Zorba the Buddha (Anthony Quinn would have done a bang-up job in the role), early Rajneesh was a shining example of eccentric, electrifying twentieth-century spiritualism. In syncretic, mischievous sermons he warned that innate human characteristics such as humor and creativity were being stifled by doctrinaire belief systems. "He had put psy-chotherapy, anarchism and religious experience together in a strik-ingly original way," wrote a follower known only as Sam in his fascinating book *Life of Osho*, a chronicle of his experiences within Rajneesh's universe. "Osho had been the closest thing the late twen-tieth century had seen to a major prophet," Sam claims.[6]

In decline, Rajneesh came across as a lurid madman, jungle crazy, like the deranged Kurtz from Joseph Conrad's novel *Heart of Darkness*. Drug-addled and pain-racked, he watched over a circus of avarice and carnality with spectacular ineptitude, unable or unwilling to corral the sublimated lusts and insatiable ids he had loosed. Toward his tawdry end Rajneesh had also become perhaps the worst judge of character in human history, surrounded by a cabal of insidious troublemakers that could be described as mere kooks—were it not for the fact that they also dabbled in a little bioterrorism.

Born into a Jain family and raised primarily by a doting grand-mother, Rajneesh was a rebellious and gifted student. Having studied philosophy at a Jain college he toured India giving lectures critical of established religions, particularly Hinduism. His later tar-gets included socialism and Gandhi; both, he said, glorified rather than rejected poverty. Rajneesh favored India's embrace of science and capitalism as a way to reverse what he saw as the country's backwardness.

Rajneesh soon capitalized on his interest in capitalism. His controversial lectures caught on, and Rajneesh was in demand as a spiritual teacher. In 1966 he went into guruship full time, leading meditation camps and offering spiritual guidance to wealthy patrons. In 1970 he began accepting Western followers, and spent most of the decade teaching at a large ashram in Pune, south of Bombay, paid for in part by his affluent patrons. From this palatial Club Meditation, Rajneesh's writings and audio and video recordings reached a worldwide audience. The yoga that Rajneesh peddled had little to do with contorting the body and everything to do with taming the mind. In his 1984 book, *Yoga: The Science of the Soul,* Rajneesh reminded followers that "when there is no mind, you are in yoga; when there is mind you are not in yoga."[7]

What Rajneesh's followers mostly got, however, was more New Age "personal growth" than traditional yoga. His ashram was a precursor to self-empowerment empires, based on teachings that echoed and supported much of the rhetoric sounded by the Human Potential movement in the West. The ashram's Encounter Group sessions, which accounted for much of its tidy income, often erupted into violence or devolved (evolved?) into fornication. A hard-to-find 1981 documentary (which I have not seen) titled *Ashram* offered a glimpse: "Scenes of these therapies have the mood of other movies' madhouse episodes," wrote Janet Maslin in her *New York Times* review. "A group pillow-fight meant to release violent instincts becomes a naked free-for-all, accompanied by the most piercing screams of fear and rage," she wrote, adding that one woman who was "very nearly raped" in the film turned out to be very content at the ashram. "The violent therapy, she says, has helped her to overcome her fear of men."[8]

Yes, there was plenty of sex at Rajneesh's ashram. In keeping with the social revolution sweeping the West, Rajneesh had for years been calling on Indians to adopt more open attitudes toward sexual matters. His followers dug this. After all, they were not your typical *sannyasis*—the Sanskrit word used to describe religious renunciates who traditionally forgo family, material goods and pleasures of the flesh. Rajneesh's neo-sannyasis swapped the ascetic for the celebratory.

"I am against all types of so-called renunciation because they are life denying, life negating and in a way anti-god," Rajneesh preached.[9]

Drugs played their obligatory part. Although Rajneesh never advocated enlightenment through drugs, a little LSD couldn't hurt either, he suggested. "LSD can only be a help to project whatsoever is in the seed form of your unconscious mind. If it is love, then love will be projected. If it is hatred, then hatred will be projected," he once said.[10] These attitudes did not endear Rajneesh to the agents of law enforcement or to the ashram's strict Hindu neighbors—especially when allegations surfaced that some of Rajneesh's followers were financing their time in India through drug running and prostitution.[11]

By most accounts the Pune ashram had become an emotionally undisciplined, orgiastic, Dionysian funhouse. In a December 1984 edition of *Newsweek,* writers Neal Karlen and Pamela Abramson quoted one of the "well-heeled Americans and Europeans drawn to his encounter therapies and free-love reputation," as the magazine described it. "A lot of people came for sex, a lot came for drugs," the ashramite said. "He offered us total freedom. It was wild." It was too wild for Richard Price, the founding therapist of the California-based Esalen Institute, the premier Human Potential center in America at the time. According to *Newsweek,* Price "renounced the movement soon after he saw a sannyasi break another disciple's arm in a therapy session."[12]

Things started to unravel toward the end of the seventies. The conservative Hindu government came down hard, denying the ashram a land-use approval for expansion, denying visas to foreign visitors who wished to visit the ashram and revoking the ashram's tax-exempt status, leaving Rajneesh owing $5 million in current and back taxes. Then there were the assassination attempts. In May 1980, during one of Rajneesh's morning discourses, a fundamentalist Hindu threw a knife at him. It clattered impotently at the guru's feet. Shortly afterward, two unexplained bombings burned part of the ashram library and a row of bicycles. Piddling affairs really, but assassination attempts are never encouraging. Under attack and with his hopes of utopian expansion dashed, Rajneesh began looking west.

The United States of Rajneesh

The guru knew how to make an entrance. Taking his first steps on United States soil in 1981, Rajneesh declared, "I am the Messiah America has been waiting for."[13] He'd ostensibly come to remedy a back problem. He was always frail, and to prevent what seemed like the inevitable deterioration of his health, one of his most ardent followers, an American-educated Indian woman named Ma Anand Sheela, wanted him to have access to the best medical care available. The group settled first in Montclair, New Jersey, and quickly picked up one follower of note: Shannon Jo Ryan, the daughter of U.S. Representative Leo Ryan, who just three years earlier had been slain by the Jonestown cult in Guyana. "If I thought there was any chance of this becoming another Jonestown, I'd run away," she told *People* magazine. "It is impossible that Bhagwan would ever ask people to kill anyone. But if he asked me to do it, I don't know. I love and trust him very much. To me he is God," Ryan said.[14] People shook their heads.

By the fall of 1981 the Rajneeshees had loaded their wagons and were moving west, toward Oregon. Their new home was a 64,000-acre, $6 million spread, paid for by Sheela. Known as Big Muddy Ranch, it was soon renamed Rancho Rajneesh. Straddling Jefferson and Wasco counties, the property lay primarily in Wasco County, population twenty thousand. It was and remains a generally traditional and overwhelmingly Christian corner of the world.

The Rajneeshees quickly began to alienate the conservative locals, who were unsettled by the group's bawdy belief system. There was the nudist camp, for one, "where commune school children and visitors are bussed in each day to join the faithful," as *Hinduism Today* magazine noted in a 1984 article.[15] The group's whole approach to childrearing probably gave locals the heebie-jeebies. "Children do not have to live with their parents or be with them: they belong to the community," reported Dialog Center International in 1982, a network that tracks new religious movements. "Some children were running around naked in the schoolhouse, and it is not unusual for boys and girls to sleep together."[16]

Naked children aside, it must be noted that the Oregon commune lacked the delirium that came to define the group's experiment in

Inner Children

English journalist Tim Guest grew up in several Rajneesh communes during the eighties. He was brought into the group at age six by his mother, a lapsed Catholic who, having surrendered herself to Rajneesh, followed the guru across three continents. Ashram children lived in communal dormitories, away from their parents. Although surrounded by other children, Guest says it was a lonely childhood and remembers going for long periods without his mother's love or guidance. In fact, children were often seen as a nuisance by the adults, who were busy indulging in all the unruly aspects of ashram life, Guest says. "It was a way for a lot of people to have a second childhood. And I think when you're having a second childhood children sort of get in the way," Guest said on New York Public Radio's *Leonard Lopate Show* in 2005.

Pune. Perhaps it was the injection of good old American puritanism, or the new specter of AIDS, a disease that bamboozled and completely terrified Rajneesh. Either way, much of the sex-soaked, drug-fueled hedonism was absent from the new ashram experience. This was about long days of hard, honest, outside work and worshipful nights full of meditation and yoga. It was the kind of functional, communal asceticism that many westerners had been so desperately seeking. It was aparigraha for Americans.

And that's perhaps what scared locals most, the group's *competence.* Within three years the Rajneeshees magically transformed a dusty valley in the Oregon high desert into a shining hippie city on a hill, a thriving, self-contained agricultural community. By far the largest spiritual society ever pioneered in America, it was serviced by an airstrip, had its own water and sewage system and featured a hotel, a shopping mall, a well-equipped hospital, a library and a casino. (How many renunciates do you know who go to casinos?) Karlen and Abramson's *Newsweek* article offered a glimpse of life at the ashram: There were forty commune businesses, "all staffed by some of the 1200 sannyasis who 'worship' at their jobs in exchange for $10 a month. Others find employment at establishments like the Rajneesh deli and pizzeria, the Rajneesh hair and beauty salon or the Rajneesh bookstore, whose stock consists entirely of the prolific Bhagwan's 350 titles."[17]

The group was run in an idiosyncratic manner, even by typical ashram standards. Rajneesh was the final authority, despite that he had little direct involvement in daily operations. In fact, having gotten to his exalted position by dint of verbal skill, Rajneesh had gone into a self-imposed silence in April 1981, eventually communicating only through Sheela, now his personal secretary. It was Sheela who outlined his plans and goals to the group, who controlled the finances, who directed most of the group's operations. In turn Sheela relied on a small cabal of mostly female functionaries, called "Moms" or "Big Moms," depending on their rank.

Sheela was accountable only to Rajneesh, and her decisions were almost always the final say. Nor did she brook opposition, an authoritarian style that made her unpopular with many Rajneeshees. She was even less popular with the locals, a strategic blunder on the Rajneeshees' part, considering that she was also the commune's public face. (*Newsweek* recounted a 1982 city-council meeting during which Sheela claimed local students looked "retarded.")[18]

Nor was Rajneesh acquitting himself well with the locals or the media. To them Rajneesh was just another money-grubbing Rasputin in an ivory tower. It was true that Rajneesh had very little contact with his followers. He spent much of his time alone or in the company of his girlfriend, an Englishwoman named Christine Woolf, known to everyone as Vivek. He rarely ventured into the ashram itself, preferring to stay sequestered in his purpose-built trailer complex, complete with an indoor swimming pool and wide-screen TV. Most followers saw their esteemed leader only when he drove by in one of his ninety-three Rolls-Royce cars. "He seemed to have turned into a caricature of self-indulgent despotism—wearing flamboyant robes and demanding more and more Rolls-Royces to add to his already huge collection," writes former follower Sam in his book *Life of Osho*. "People said he was on drugs. At times it seemed almost as though he was deliberately trying to look like a charlatan."[19] It was not the aparigraha we'd come to expect from our gurus.

(The Rolls-Royce also happens to be Bikram Choudhury's status symbol of choice. Rollers were the Indian maharajas' favorite cars during British colonial rule. The nizam of Hyderabad boasted a fifty-strong fleet. Rolls-Royce halted shipment of cars to the continent in the mid-fifties and returned only in 2005, lured back by India's new moneyed elite. If there'd been more Rollers around when Osho and Bikram were boys, maybe their followers would have been saved a lot of bother and expense.)

Greed Is God

"Jesus Saves, Moses Invests, Bhagwan Spends"

—a popular bumper sticker seen around the Rajneesh ashram

The real turning point in relations between the locals and the Rajneeshees came in May 1982, when the group seized control of a small town near the ashram called Antelope. As a way of getting around the stringent land-use laws that constrained the commune's expansion efforts, and as they had grown larger in number than the inhabitants of the town, the Rajneeshees voted to incorporate their commune. Overnight the new city of Rajneeshpuram was created, effectively annexing Antelope. The group created a police department it called the "Peace Force," a concept George Orwell surely dreamed up. Having their own cops made the group's already bellicose attitude toward self-defense even more alarming. *Oregon Magazine,* which ran many investigative pieces on the commune, reported that the group could defend itself with "AR-15s, CAR-15s and Uzi Model Bs" guns—from a stockpile of weapons larger than all Oregon's police departments combined.[20]

Paranoia was increasingly in style. By summer 1984 Sheela had secretly installed electronic surveillance equipment throughout the commune.[21] At the same time, Rajneesh's vision of the future was becomingly increasingly bleak. In 1984 he predicted that two-thirds of humanity would die from AIDS. He also predicted that a nuclear holocaust would destroy humankind sometime in the 1990s.[22] (Whew!) But the Rajneeshees had reasons to be paranoid since the U.S. Attorney's office in Portland, Oregon, had taken charge of an immigration investigation regarding sham marriages at the commune.

Then came an Oregon Court of Appeals decision that invalidated the town of Rajneeshpuram's charter. The Rajneeshees' only hope for a new incorporation was through the Wasco County court. Two of the three elected commissioners were seen as virulently anticommune, but all three commissioners were facing re-election in November, just a few weeks hence. Some desperate action would be required to sway the election—action so desperate that it became the twentieth century's only successful bioterrorism attack on American soil.

Sects Crime

The Dalles is a small farm town on the banks of the Columbia River, about eighty-five miles east of Portland. It's the seat of Wasco's county, and a quiet, peaceful place. Or had been anyway—until September 1984, when over seven hundred of the town's ten thousand residents became violently ill after eating in local restaurants. It was an outbreak of *Salmonella typhimurium,* a common strain of the salmonella bacteria that causes nausea and vomiting, often accompanied by diarrhea, fever, chills, headache and fainting.

The Dalles salmonella outbreak came in two waves, about ten days apart. The first wave began September 10 and was comparatively mild, accounting for about 100 reported cases. The second wave began September 21—and soon filled to capacity the Mid-Columbia Medical Center, the local hospital. Confused, frightened patients waited in hallways as overworked doctors scrambled to treat more than 600 cases. The county eventually confirmed 751 cases of salmonella poisoning. Although there were no fatalities, more than 45 people were hospitalized and another 117 residents showed severe symptoms. A pregnant woman with symptoms gave birth to a baby who also showed effects of the poison.

The outbreak was highly unusual, particularly since The Dalles had not had a single case of salmonella poisoning in six years before the outbreak. Then health authorities uncovered one important common denominator: Most victims had eaten from the salad bar at one of eight restaurants implicated in the outbreak. (Two restaurants without salad bars were also implicated, though fewer cases were reported in these restaurants.) And another significant clue: Salmonella was found in these restaurants' salad dressings but not in the mix used to make the dressing, suggesting a contamination had happened after the mix had been made.

Democratic Congressman Jim Weaver, who represented Oregon's 4th District in Congress from 1975 to 1987, suspected the Rajneeshees and said as much in a speech to the United States House of Representatives. Weaver became an enemy of the Rajneeshees early on, when he'd stymied a land-swap deal between the Rajneeshees and the federal government that would have allowed the group to build a large resort and housing development. On February 28, 1985, he came at them head-on. "Who would want to do it [the poisoning]? And who would have the capability to do it?" Weaver asked the house. He focused his suspicion on Ma Anand Sheela, Rajneesh's right-hand mom, quoting from a newspaper report in which she allegedly claimed that Wasco County was "so bigoted it deserves to be taken over." He explained that the Rajneeshees had a "well equipped medical laboratory" at Rajneeshpuram. But most damning was the story he recounted of the two county commissioners considered hostile to the Rajneeshees who became violently ill, exhibiting symptoms of salmonella poisoning, after visiting the commune on county business and accepting cups of water from the Rajneeshees.[23]

In 1999 Dr. Seth Carus, deputy director of the Center for the Study of Weapons of Mass Destruction, authored a working paper titled *Bioterrorism and Biocrimes: The Illicit Use of Biological Agents in the 20th Century.* The paper, based on court records, interviews and media reports, offers perhaps the best summation of the Rajneesh poisoning plot. Its most important source was a man named Krishna Deva (born David Berry Knapp), the mayor of Rajneeshpuram at the time of the poisonings and a confidant of Ma Anand Sheela who eventually turned state's evidence. According to Knapp, the plot was spearheaded by Sheela and carried out by half a dozen crazies. Chief among this rogues' gallery was a nasty piece of work named Ma Anand Puja. Born Diane Ivonne Onang in the Philippines and raised in California, Puja joined the commune in 1979. Trained as a nurse, she soon became director of the ashram's health center and secretary-treasurer of the Rajneesh Medical Corporation, giving her authority over the center's pharmacy and clinic. Puja might have been a "Big Mom" but there was little maternal love for her. Described as a loner and a tyrant (ashramites called her Doctor Mengele behind her back), Puja "delighted in death, poisons and the idea of carrying out various plots," according to Knapp.[24]

This modern-day Lucrezia Borgia also had a positively spine-chilling obsession with AIDS. "Puja talked about culturing the AIDS virus and she was very secretive concerning her work in that area," Knapp claimed. Puja may have deliberately infected at least one person to see if it was possible for her to transmit the HIV virus, according to an FBI agent's unconfirmed allegation.[25] And Puja, in concert with Sheela, may have been involved in the June 1980 death of Sheela's first husband, Chinmaya, who was sick with Hodgkin's disease. In her book, *The Promise of Paradise,* former Rajneesh follower Satya Bharti Franklin writes that Sheela told Knapp in 1985 she had injected Chinmaya with one of Puja's poisons the night of his death.[26] Euthanizing a gravely ill, possibly willing patient would have been child's play, compared with what the Toxic Twins had cooked up for the residents of Wasco County.

Sheela was determined to sway the county commissioner elections at any cost. One ploy was the implausibly bizarre Share-a-Home scheme, which involved trucking hundreds of homeless down-and-outers from around the country into the commune, supposedly to offer food and housing to their new friends. The ulterior motive was to register all the homeless to vote—and to induce them into voting for the Rajneeshees' preferred candidate. Another plot, according to Knapp, involved putting pathogens (specifically, dead rodents) into the Wasco County water system.[27] And at some point—likely with Puja's fevered input—it was decided that sickening county residents would be an effective method to lessen turnout. The logic was simple: A voter who was retching his or her insides out was unlikely to go to the polls.

Puja had a few bio-tricks up her sleeve. One was *Salmonella typhi,* the organism that causes typhoid fever, which Puja was said to favor because victims would suffer weeks of fever. She also expressed interest in the hepatitis virus. In the end Puja eschewed the flashy and went with the tried and true, another strain of salmonella called *Salmonella enterica typhimurium,* which she obtained from a commercial supplier. She cooked up her witches' brew in a well-appointed laboratory secreted away deep within the recesses of the ashram.[28] (Residents of earth should breathe a sigh of relief that her AIDS-transmission fixation never got off the ground.)

A few test runs followed; in August 1984 the Rajneeshees gave salmonella-spiked water to two county commissioners, the attack congressman Weaver cited in his speech before congress. They spread salmonella-spiked liquid on doorknobs and urinal handles in the Wasco County courthouse. Their final test was the most fun. Puja and Sheela sprinkled their "salsa," as they called it, on produce in a local supermarket in order to give shoppers "the shits." Afterward, "Puja was giggling and saying that she had a good time," Knapp recalled. By September 1984 Sheela and her cronies couldn't help themselves—and poured the remaining vials of salmonella on salad bars at restaurants throughout The Dalles.[29] The rest is bio-terrorism history.

The Rajneeshees ultimately failed in their attempt to swing the election. The success of the restaurant contamination had the counterproductive consequence of bringing sudden publicity to the town, making any further salsa shenanigans almost impossible. And when county officials heard that an estimated four thousand homeless people might have been brought in to sway the election, they declared that every new voter would have to be interviewed before registration. (As a result, the Rajneeshees spat most of this suddenly useless human debris, with no return tickets, food or lodging, back out into the surrounding communities, overwhelming services organizations. So much for new friends.)

With their crackpot plot having come to zilch, commune leaders now urged their followers to boycott the election, although that was most likely a face-saving move. On November 9, 1984, *The New York Times* reported that between Rajneesh disciples and the remaining homeless people living at the commune, the group could muster only 239 votes.[30] It would be nice to think, although there's no evidence for it, that there was a general apathy among rank-and-file Rajneeshees toward provincial revolution. Anyway, it was too late to play nice. By then the whole town had the shits.

Why didn't someone with a shred of moral fiber put an end to these Jacobean turns? And where was Rajneesh? What did he know and when did he know it? According to David Knapp, in the report of an interview conducted by the Oregon attorney general's office, Sheela said "she had talked with Bhagwan about the plot to decrease voter turnout in The Dalles by making people sick. Sheela said that Bhagwan commented that it was best not to hurt people, but if a few died not to worry."[31] Rajneesh later denied any involvement in the attacks. He certainly never implicated himself—although not from a lack of opportunities. In her campaign to eavesdrop on every inch of Rajneeshpuram, Sheela made sure to bug Rajneesh's room especially well. God knows what secrets were plucked from inside that mystic boudoir, but no evidence of the guru's involvement in Sheela's harebrained schemes was ever offered.

Then again, what would Rajneesh know? He'd spent much of the previous few years—I'm not making this up—sitting in a dentist's chair, getting high. Naturally, this was a flagrant violation of the commune's stringent no-drugs policy. Rajneesh's former bodyguard, Hugh Milne, in his book *Bhagwan: The God That Failed,* recounts the time he was asked to photograph Rajneesh in his dental chair for posterity. (It was from this chair that Rajneesh allegedly dictated three of his bestselling books, all while high as a kite.) There was Rajneesh, surrounded by his dentist, dental assistant, personal physician and girlfriend, Vivek, calmly taking hits from a bottle of nitrous oxide as the assistant wrote down everything Rajneesh said. "I noticed that everybody in the room apart from me seemed to be completely unaffected by what was going on. They were obviously all used to it," Milne wrote. While it was mostly dopey brain-droppings coming out of Rajneesh's mouth, Milne's esteemed leader did say something so provocative that it eventually motivated Milne to leave the commune: "I am so relieved that I do not have to pretend to be enlightened any more," the great guru let slip.[32]

Waiting to Exhale

Rajneesh ended his three-and-a-half-year vow of public silence on October 30, 1984, in the lead-up to the Wasco County elections. In retrospect, Rajneesh's return to full voice can be seen as a careful and well-orchestrated pre-emptive strike, preparation for a day when he might have to throw the Moms under the bus. That bus arrived a little less than a year later, on September 16, 1985. Rajneesh had called a press conference, and, boy, was it a doozy, even by his standards. His first dramatic announcement to the salivating press corps was that Sheela, Puja and a dozen others had fled the commune for Europe. "I have brought you media people here to inform you of the glad news that this commune is free from a fascist regime," Rajneesh continued. "Adolf Hitler has died again." Rajneesh also claimed that Sheela had absconded with roughly $50 million of the ashram's money. The media had a field day, painting the kind of "mad cult" articles we've been gobbling up for over one hundred years. "Departed Aides Accused by Guru of Murder Attempts, Theft of Millions," screamed the *Los Angeles Times*.[33] (One can only imagine the delight editors felt at getting the words *guru* and *murder* in the same headline.)

In the string of public press conferences that followed, Rajneesh blamed Sheela and the Gang for an astounding litany of offenses: the salmonella attacks, the land grabs, the bugging of the commune, the attempted contamination of The Dalles water system, not to mention the attempted poisonings of Rajneesh's physician, dentist and girlfriend, as well as the attempted murder of neighboring Jefferson County's district attorney. Rajneesh begged the authorities to investigate his claims, and they did so—sluggishly. There seemed to be the sense that Rajneesh had to be padding Sheela's exotic résumé of offenses. "I don't think all the cards are face up on the table yet," Oregon attorney general Dave Frohnmayer said at the time.[34] Rajneesh claimed that investigators were more intent on bringing *him* down than capturing the bad guys. "We have given them solid proofs, and they have not taken a single step," he said. "They want to commit a bigger crime: Their interest is in destroying the commune."[35]

Investigators eventually made their move. On October 2, 1985, fifty law enforcement officers entered the ranch and ransacked Puja's clandestine germ-warfare kitchen, where they found glass vials containing the implicated salmonella strain, an assortment of other bio-nasties and a copy of *The Anarchist Cookbook,* an instruction manual for the production of homemade explosives and eavesdropping devices that is widely read among nut-jobs. The investigation would drag on for years, uncovering a string of insane narratives: The commune had arranged more than four hundred sham marriages, some Rajneeshees had plotted to kill Charles Turner, U.S. attorney general for Oregon at the time, in order to stop an immigration investigation;[36] and one fool even came forward to confess his part in a plan to crash a plane loaded with bombs into a Wasco County courthouse.[37]

On October 23, 1985, a federal grand jury issued a thirty-five-count indictment charging Rajneesh, Sheela and other disciples with conspiracy to evade immigration laws. There was talk of cops taking Rajneesh by force. Tensions peaked. The tide had turned, and some redder-necked locals now apparently grew giddy with thoughts of revenge. "Threats and demands that Bhagwan and his sannyasis leave the country poured in," wrote Sue Appleton, a Rajneesh apologist. "There was a definite feeling of a lynching in the offing."[38] The Oregon National Guard and State Police were called in, but nobody was making any fast moves. Just how many guns the commune had was anyone's guess, and the word *Jonestown* was ringing in everybody's ears.

Rajneesh's solution was ingeniously simple: He ran away. On October 27, 1985, Rajneesh, his physician, housekeeper, cook and a few followers chartered a Learjet bound for Bermuda, taking with them a .38 revolver, Teflon-coated ammunition, $58,522 in currency and $1 million in jewelry. On its way to sunnier climes, the jet stopped at Charlotte Douglas International Airport in North Carolina. That's when federal agents swooped, arresting Rajneesh on suspicion of trying to escape charges of immigration fraud. Most of his sannyasis didn't even know he'd fled until they heard media reports of his arrest.

That same day in West Germany, FBI agents accompanied by German federal police arrested Sheela and Puja. They were extradited to Portland in February 1986 to face federal and state charges of attempted murder, first- and second-degree assault, product tampering (for the salmonella poisonings), wiretapping and immigration offenses. Sheela was sentenced to sixty-four years. Puja received forty-five years. After serving just twenty-nine months of their sentences in a minimum-security federal prison in California, the Poison Pals were released early for good behavior. Sheela skedaddled back to Europe to avoid state charges and remains a fugitive. She started life again as—no kidding—the administrator of a nursing home for mentally disabled patients. "The same love I had for people at Rajneeshpuram, I bring to my patients now," she told the *Willamette Week,* a Portland-based alternative weekly, in 2004.[39] Let's just hope patients are drinking bottled water. No one seems to know where Puja ended up. I can't help thinking of the last scene from the film *Silence of the Lambs,* as escaped killer Hannibal Lecter fades quietly into the crowd.

Rajneesh's downfall was a full-throated media circus with its own cinematic dimension. Rajneesh's mug was splashed across every newspaper in America as cops dragged him in chains from North Carolina to the Oklahoma City jail. From there he gave a live jailhouse interview to Ted Koppel on ABC's *Nightline,* a groggy performance that must have seemed to viewers like a scene from some Bizarro World, all-guru version of the classic heist film *Dog Day Afternoon.* In the original, bank robber Al Pacino negotiates a plane to fly him and his partner-in-crime to another country—beyond the jurisdiction of American law. He then has to deny his partner's first choice of Wyoming because "Wyoming's not a country." In the guru version, Rajneesh tells a dubious Koppel he was not fleeing arrest or leaving the country by heading to the Bahamas because he thought Bermuda was just another American state.[40]

Rajneesh was shipped back to Oregon to face charges of criminal conspiracy, thirty-four counts of making false statements to federal officials and two counts of immigration fraud. At first Rajneesh pleaded not guilty to all the charges but, as part of a deal his lawyers made, later changed his plea to no contest to two lesser charges, one of making false statements and one of conspiracy. Investigators never found sufficient evidence to link Rajneesh to any of the commune's biggest crimes. In the end, getting him on immigration violations was like getting Al Capone on tax evasion and not murder, but it was something. His lawyer cut a deal. Rajneesh was given a ten-year suspended sentence and placed on five years' probation. In addition, he agreed to pay $400,000 in fines and prosecution costs. Most significantly, at least symbolically, he agreed to leave the United States. By dinnertime the next day, the guru was gone. Author Christopher Hitchens tartly summed up the situation in his book *God Is Not Great*: "I would say that the people of Antelope, Oregon, missed being as famous as Jonestown by a fairly narrow margin."[41]

The commune itself quickly became a ghost town. Shell-shocked sannyasis packed up their belongings and wondered whom to follow next. Oregon's drenching November rains turned the land back into what it had been when the Rajneeshees first arrived, a big muddy ranch. Eventually, the ranch was sold at auction and is now owned by the Young Life Christian ministry (uh-oh), which has converted it into a youth camp called Wildhorse Canyon. Let's pray their kitchen is far away from Puja's germ-warfare lab. In Antelope a small plaque was placed at the base of the post-office flagpole to commemorate the tiny town surviving its short-lived conquest. It reads, "Dedicated to those of this community who through the Rajneesh invasion and occupation of 1981–85 remained, resisted and remembered."

The rest of Rajneesh's life was ramshackle. Although physically frail, he embarked on a "world tour" immediately after his ejection from the United States that became dismal when twenty-one countries denied him entry. He returned to India in July 1986 and was back at his old ashram in Pune by January 1987. He continued making pronouncements that alternated between wise and weird. In November 1987 he claimed his failing health was because of poison that American authorities had administered when he was held in custody.[42] A year later he announced he would no longer answer to "Bhagwan Shree Rajneesh" and had instead taken the moniker "Osho," meaning friend or teacher. In early 1989 he was floating the idea of moving his whole operation to what was still the Soviet Union. The goal was to fuse his autocratic mysticism with the USSR's atheistic Communism—despite that Mikhail Gorbachev's perestroika was rapidly moving the country toward capitalism.

On December 9, 1989, just two days before a big celebration for what was to be Rajneesh's fifty-eighth birthday, his girlfriend was found dead in a Bombay hotel room. Few facts are known about Vivek's life, let alone her death. "The story was that it was a drug overdose—but whether accidental or a deliberate decision to kill herself, no one knew. In fact, no one knew whether she did really die in Bombay—or whether it was in the ashram, and they just hushed it up. Whatever it was, she seems to have been in a state of great inner pain," recounts Sam in his book *Life of Osho*. "She was his lover, and the only friend he ever had. She gave everything she had, and I think it tore her apart."[43] Osho died less than seven weeks later, on January 19, 1990, at age fifty-eight, of heart failure. His ashes are enshrined at the Pune ashram. An epitaph reads, "OSHO. Never Born, Never Died. Only Visited this Planet Earth."

I will surely be accused of giving Rajneesh short shrift here as a spiritual leader. There's no doubt that he was a highly original religious thinker. For over twenty years he was able to bind together non sequiturs from a stunning array of topics into spontaneous, eloquent spiritual oratory that engendered utter devotion in his followers. That alone should be evidence enough of his powers as a mystical chieftain. But the sad fact is that the Grand Guignol Rajneesh allowed to occur on his watch has greatly and rightly overshadowed his spiritual legacy.

And ... Release!

It's easy to explain the wayward actions of die-hard followers: They behave the way they think their gurus want them to. It would be a facile argument were it not so often true. Figuring out what drives the gurus, that's trickier. And if the Rajneesh story teaches us anything, it's that greed comes in many forms. It's easy to get steamed at mega-rich mystics, but the most egregious breaches of aparigraha often have little to do with material concerns. Gurus deal in the currency of devotion and control. How committed are you? Are you willing to give up not just your possessions but everything you've held dear? Your community, your friends, in some cases even your family? It's no surprise that ashrams are full of mostly the young, single and childless. They're the ones the gurus go after. Unattached devotees are loose with their wallets, focused on their (i.e., the ashram's) work and much more devoted; they're less apt to put others (like those damn kids) before themselves. The desire for childless disciples often takes an aggressive form: There may be a demand for sexual abstinence. In extreme cases, women have been persuaded to abort pregnancies and men encouraged to undergo sterilization. Mistakes happen, though, and children sometimes do pop up. Some groups have been known to take children away from birth parents to be raised by another (or every) member of the group. If you ask me, breaking up families in order to increase pliancy among followers is an act of despicable greed. But that's just me.

Family bonds certainly weren't very strong around the SYDA ashram, it seems. By 1981 seventy-three-year-old Swami Muktananda, the movement's scandal-plagued elder statesman, was looking for someone to replace him as guru. He made his announcement in

Unborn to Be Wild

Journalist Tim Guest describes abortions and sterilizations as "routine" procedures at the Rajneeshpuram's medical center. "The ashram was seen as not a very appropriate place for children, I think with good reason. So the message went out, indirectly, from Bhagwan that if you were pregnant and weren't ready for a child, having an abortion was okay. And if you wanted to free your energy to move sexually, being sterilized was also okay," Guest said on New York Public Radio's *Leonard Lopate Show* in 2005.

July of that year: An eighteen-year-old male monk named Nityananda would be handed the reins. Nityananda also happens to be the brother of SYDA's spiritual leader, Gurumayi, who was then known simply as Malti Shetty. The news came as a shock to most ashramites, given that Malti was considered by just about everyone to be the prime candidate. Then, just months before his death, Muktananda changed his decree to include Malti as official cosuccessor, for reasons that were never made entirely clear. You'll recall the whirlwind of carnal aches and exertions that characterized Muktananda's final years, making a mockery of his vows of brahmacharya. Now he'd handed the reins over to someone whose staggering lust for control would make her vow of aparigraha all but irrelevant.

Although many people suspected Gurumayi's power-sharing agreement with her brother was doomed to failure, no one could have predicted the familial power struggle of mafia proportions that was to come. Journalist Lis Harris elaborated on this preposterous chain of events in an excellent article she wrote for the November 1994 issue of *The New Yorker* titled "O Guru, Guru, Guru." According to Harris, Nityananda was content to let his sister essentially run the ashram. Even so, in late 1985, during a visit to the Indian SYDA ashram, several members of Gurumayi's staff accosted Nityananda, shouting at him that he'd been stripped of his power as a guru. Nityananda tried to flee but was told the tires on all the ashram cars had been slashed. Nityananda confronted Gurumayi in person—and again found himself surrounded. For the next eighteen days, Harris says, he was held as a virtual prisoner in a small room at the ashram and berated daily by Gurumayi's goons.

It didn't end there. A few days later Gurumayi convened a group of followers that included four women Nityananda admitted to having (consensual) sex with. At Gurumayi's insistence, the group struck Nityananda with a bamboo cane—*for three hours.* "At one point she [Gurumayi] said, 'Maybe I should beat him on his penis. That's the cause of all this,' " Nityananda told Harris. Admitting later to the incident, Gurumayi claimed her brother received only a few slaps from the four women, "in addition to a few slaps from me."

At the end of 1985 SYDA officials announced that Nityananda would be relinquishing his role as cosuccessor and guru because his term had expired. Five months later SYDA made another announcement: The *real* reason for Nityananda's stepping down was that he'd broken his vow of celibacy. In fact, he'd broken his vow six times, as he admitted to Harris. But in Nityananda's opinion, the reason he was ousted from SYDA has nothing to do with sex. It was greed. "I just think she [Gurumayi] wanted the whole thing for herself, and she tried to come up with a way to do it—to have the whole organization, the devotees, the money, the power as a guru, solely, without having to share or have anything to do with me," he says.[44] So much for family.

Symbolically and mentally stripped, Nityananda eventually made a public announcement that he was no longer a guru, signing papers that officially relinquished his power as co–ecclesiastical head. The final humiliation for Nityananda was his removal from SYDA's collective memory, an event former Gurumayi-follower Dan Shaw remembers well. "Like in Stalin's Russia," he says, "hundreds of his [Nityananda's] devotees sitting in a room, cutting his pictures out of magazines and books and deleting him from history."

For Shaw the whole debacle was further proof that he needed to get out. By 1992 he'd spent over a decade being pushed around by Gurumayi and her greedy gang. "I was getting pretty psychologically battered by Gurumayi in the last six months," he says. "She told me I couldn't do anything right. She told me I had no creativity, she said I was like an animal, I had a heart of stone, I'd never given anything to the ashram. She said many things that I took to heart because she was my god." It was only after gradual separation from ashram life—and two years of therapy—that the reality began to dawn on him. "This had been a crazy sick system. I bought into it, and I didn't want to see how cruel and destructive it really was," he says. Since leaving SYDA Shaw has obtained a master's degree in social work and has his own psychotherapy practice in New York. He often speaks out about the role of the guru, and his assessment is blunt. "They are parasites! They create in the follower a sense of dependence, which then allows them to parasitically exploit everything they can out of the person. And then when the person is used up they usually get tossed."

Big Yoga

Of course, there are many people in the yoga business who don't want to hear these kinds of stories. That's all in the past, they say. Things don't work that way anymore. The days of the greedy gurus are over. In some ways that's true. Rajneeshees often like to claim that his downfall was the result of a vendetta spearheaded by Ronald Reagan's government. They may have been partly right. Just as video killed the radio star, Reagan's sweeping conservatism did kill off many cultural vestiges of the flower power and New Age generations. The times, they were a-changin' back. And as the nineties dawned, yoga would be redefined again, this time as body engineering. The aged Indian swamis gave way to telegenic, homegrown Power yoga gurus. The era of Big Yoga had begun. A gleaming, corporate, streamlined one-size-fits-all industry has evolved that somehow has its finger in everything from realigning your "center" to whitening your teeth. It's the yoga of high-end resorts and spa treatments. Call them cashrams, if you will. (Ironically, one of the best examples is the Osho International Meditation Resort, as Rajneesh's ashram in Pune is now called. The center has become an established and mainstream fixture on the New Religions circuit, attracting over 200,000 visitors every year. What would Rajneesh make of this straight-up, for-profit model, the Rajneesh of 1971, who was heard telling a Japanese follower that "meditation must not be made into a business"?)[45]

One victim in all of yoga's constant upsizing would seem to be aparigraha. Yoga's roots in renunciation have become increasingly de-emphasized as the practice grows ever more glitzy. Baron Baptiste has no problem hiding his success, perhaps because he interprets it as inevitable: "I believe that if you're yogic, there's no choice, you will be successful. If you're living the yogic path, you will be successful, it's not an option." Anyway, it's not about *what* you reap, according to James Barkan, it's how. And why. "If your intention is to just make money and take advantage of people, then it's a karmic thing that is going to work against you. If your intention is to help as many people as you can, and if mass-marketing will get the word out to the masses, then I don't see anything wrong with it," he says. Rodney Yee agrees. "Why not making a living about something that you're just really impassioned about?" he asks. Adds Jivamukti cofounder Sharon Gannon, "I don't see any problem with generating money as a source of energy if it's used wisely."

But whatever happened to the hopelessly naive notion that this sort of mystical wisdom should be free? Jivamukti cofounder David Life says it's just that: naive. "The traditional yoga is you pay all you have to the guru. You scrape together every last cent you can get and you put yourself at the mercy of the teacher. Due to ignorance and unfamiliarity and also programming, westerners have a different idea about the circuit it should take." In reality, present-day yogis do have it easy. In the past seekers had to work much harder for their spiritual guidance. Potential students were expected to do years of metaphysical hard work at the feet of the master before being accepted as apprentices, if they ever were. This expression of commitment, the idea that one had to give in order to get, is almost entirely absent from the modern yoga and meditation scene. All we do is pony up the money—and complain when the money is too much. "It's ignorance that people think spirituality can exist without material or commercial elements. It can't," asserts Yoga Works founder Alan Finger. "That material center has to be stable for anything to work—for spirituality to work efficiently. We need a stable financial base and we don't want to be scared of it and we don't want to hide it. Hiding it is the problem."

Hiding his success has never been Bikram's problem. In fact, it's what has gotten him so much terrible press. That and the yoga copyright case, which has sent legions of blogging yogis ("blogis"?) into paroxysms about Bikram's lack of aparigraha. "Human greed knows no boundaries," commented one blogger on the Tao of Cheese website.[46] "Hate, ego, materialism, greed will only get you a ticket to diseaseland," wrote another person in response to a *Mother Jones* article about the case.[47] "The most serious violation he's committed is of aparigraha (greedlessness)," wrote another blogger on the Associated Content website. "He is a joke, and he has made a mockery of yoga."[48] None of this seems to bother Bikram much. It's right in line with his shtick as the humble Indian yogi who came west to beat us at our own game. "When in Rome, do as the Romans do. You have to protect your intellectual property by making copyrights, trademarks and franchising, so I did," Bikram explained to the Reuters news agency in 2008.[49]

The irony is that Bikram may have the last laugh, at least from a PR standpoint. Open Source Yoga Unity (OSYU), the group made up of yoga teachers and studios owners targeted by Bikram for copyright and trademark infringements, immediately made friends in the yoga community with its decision to resist Bikram's aggressive claims. Jim Harrison, OSYU's crusading attorney, said the case pivots on an essential question: "Can someone copyright yoga? And if you can, what protections do you have under it? We can't really walk away from this without that resolved."

But as the case drags on, OSYU's motives appear to be less and less pure. In December 2003 OSYU filed an abuse-of-copyright claim against Bikram and asked a federal court for a declaratory judgment. OSYU hopes the court will declare Bikram's claimed copyright and trademark as unenforceable. But in April 2005, in the landmark ruling, federal judge Phyllis Hamilton declared that Bikram's yoga *has* been designed in a manner creative enough to warrant protection. Writing that it seems "inappropriate, and almost unbelievable, that a sequence of yoga positions could be any one person's intellectual property," Hamilton goes on to say that the court nonetheless finds OSYU "has provided no persuasive authority" to the contrary.[50] Hamilton also dismisses the copyright-abuse claims, saying Bikram is well within his rights to enforce copyright protection.

The case is headed to trial—until OSYU instigates a settlement. Studios owners such as the McCauleys agree to stop using the Bikram name. Bikram agrees to stop litigation against them. The David and Goliath battle is over. But those watching the case are far from satisfied, believing the studio owners have put their private legal and financial concerns before that of the larger yoga community. "I thought that it was a disappointment and a betrayal of the position that they had taken," *Eweek.com* technology editor John

Pallatto, who has followed the case closely, tells me. Pallatto also wrote a column for *Eweek.com* that sharply rebuked the group. "OSYU has apparently abandoned any pretense of battling for the common good," he wrote. "OSYU's apparently altruistic act of draping itself with the mantle of the open source movement now seems crafty and disingenuous. The true state of matters has emerged and it's just business as usual."[51] The majority of yogis blogging about the outcome share Pallatto's assessment. "It is like this suit never even happened," says one.[52] "It rather creates the impression that the OSYU 'collective' was just a few studio owners who were out for themselves," says another.[53]

Citing a confidentiality clause in the settlement, the McCauleys will no longer discuss the case with me. Nor will attorney Jim Harrison. In an email declining to be interviewed, Harrison instead directs me to a released statement which says that the parties have reached a mutually satisfactory resolution. Less than a year earlier Harrison had been advocating for legal clarity, telling me this was "an area of law that needs to be adjudicated."

In Florida James Barkan *is* willing to discuss the case, but only in general terms, also citing the confidentiality clause. He gives three reasons for the settlement: "It was getting very expensive, very costly. Two, it was extremely stressful for everyone involved. And three was to just let this thing be done with." I ask him about the criticism that OSYU sold out. He responds with the group's party line: "Our purpose was not to protect ourselves. The reason we got together in the first place was to protect everybody else. And we could have sold out long ago and been indemnified and that's the last thing we wanted to do." Yet that's exactly what they eventually did. Plus, the settlement protects only OSYU members. So, after all this time and acrimony, studio owners outside the case are still scratching their heads, left to guess at what their rights and responsibilities might be. "It would have been nice to see whether a court upheld Bikram Yoga's copyrights. I think there was a strong argument to be made that they could not be enforced," Pallatto says. As it stands now, the basic copyright issues remain unresolved. And studio owners may still find themselves in Bikram's crosshairs. "The ball is in Bikram Yoga's court. If they want to pursue it against other practitioners who are trying to do similar things, they're free to press their copyright claims against them."

Bikram's reputation, meanwhile, remains more or less intact. He's still the Bad Boy of yoga. And it continues to make him tons of money.

EPILOGUE

People are so skillful in their ignorance!
—PARAMAHANSA YOGANANDA, QUOTED IN
J. DONALD WALTERS, *THE PATH: ONE MAN'S QUEST
ON THE ONLY PATH THERE IS*

In chapter 2 of the Yoga Sutras, Patanjali offers a dire warning about the five yamas. These restraints, he wrote, only fulfill their promise as a great vow when they are followed to the letter and are "not conditioned by class, place, time or occasion." In other words, for this whole yoga thing to work, one must practice the yamas everywhere, all the time. Now, far be it from me to suggest Patanjali's antediluvian fundamentalism as the ideal for space-age yogis. I offer this morsel merely as a reminder of just how strongly the "father of yoga" felt about strict adherence to principles. It also happens to be a jolting coda to our journey through the business, the ethical minefield, if you will, of yoga.

So, you may be wondering, where does all this leave us? Is it possible to selectively interpret the ethics intrinsic to yoga and still be a true yogi? Or is selective interpretation the only way for modern men and women to meet yoga's high moral standard? Does yoga's underlying philosophy grow in stature under the gaze of relativism or does it crumble apart? We needn't answer right away. Yoga isn't going anywhere. We have simply come to need it too much. And people may need it even more during the tough times that may be ahead. "Job stress, job loss, family problems, money problems. They need some sanctuary for their soul. And yoga provides that," says economic consultant and futurist Barry Minkin. "All of us are looking for answers. We are looking for the great truth," says cult specialist Rick Ross. "We want someone to give us the answers, perhaps instantly in Western culture, where we're used to drive-throughs and microwaves. And now we think we can get instant enlightenment."

But will yoga continue its Teflon trajectory through the popular culture? Can it continue to veer between the sacred and profane without its much-ballyhooed good karma eventually coming undone? "Can yoga survive all this commercialization, industrialization and so on? Yes, absolutely. It has been around five thousand years. It teaches the truth, and nothing can touch that ever," says Trisha Lamb.

"I do think that there are levels of engagement. And it may be that we are engaging at the most superficial level of yoga right now," says author Stefanie Syman. "But I don't think anything about yoga has been 'lost.'" Barnaby Harris proclaims, "It's not like it's going to burn itself out. It's made it this far. It's a good product that will survive whatever this is." Others are less cavalier. Barry Minkin believes the endless repackaging of yoga can't continue forever. He imagines a day when "some movie star or somebody who people see as a representative … stands up against some of these practices and says, 'This is wrong, this is not what yoga is about.'" The increasing elitism of yoga, meanwhile, concerns Yoga Works cofounder George Lichter. "I see the affluence connected to yoga, and that doesn't feel right to me," he says.

We can take comfort, if that's the word for it, from the fact that yoga is by no means the only spiritual or philosophical system to become grist for the capitalist mill. Sacred Hindu images such as Lord Ganesha have found themselves on designer toilet seats and women's shoes. In the sacred city of Mecca, a new shopping mall filled with fast food, Starbucks and lingerie shops now literally overshadows Islam's holiest site, the Al-Masjid al-Haram. And the number of Jesus-inspired hip-hop clothing labels alone boggles the mind. ("Christ First," "Righteouz Gear" and "Sonz of God" are among my favorites.) Yet followers continue to wring meaning from these battered traditions. Yoga is no different, says Amrit Desai. "People who have spiritual awakening and who are real seekers will find the real path out of it anyway," he says. "I'm just excited that the right people will find something very beautiful that yoga has to offer." Rodney Yee believes we could all benefit from a wider view. "I think the yoga practice in the United State is actually really healthy," he says. "It's all fun and games in some ways. I mean, we have to take ourselves a little less seriously." The final word—and take it for what it's worth—belongs to renowned yogi Alan Finger. "I really think it's all as it should be," he says. "The universe is behind this, not us. And so yoga will go exactly where it needs to go."

It's worth noting what's happened to some of the people I've met during the making of the documentary and subsequent writing of this book. After closing her New York City studio, Marilyn Barnett returned home to Arizona, where she went back to work as a registered nurse. Although she regularly practices yoga, she no longer teaches. Barnett's former business partner, Anne Libby, also left the business and teaches now only as a volunteer. She also counsels small-business owners in what she calls the "yoga of small business." The yoga studio opened by Barnett's former teacher in her and Libby's old space has since gone out of business.

By the time of our last interview, Trisha Lamb had already quit her job as media liaison for the Yoga Research and Education Center. Shortly after we spoke, she entered a three-year silent (as in no speaking) Buddhist retreat. Her goal was to eventually be meditating twenty-four hours a day.

In addition to running the Academia de Yoga in San Jose del Cabo, Mexico, Tony Sanchez is now director of yoga for a string of resort hotels. His former studio in San Francisco has become a striptease school.

It took him a while, but Barnaby Harris eventually crafted a follow up to "Fuck Yoga" and began printing "Fuck Frank Gehry" T-shirts. The ironic power of the shirt was undercut, however, when

Gehry himself decided to get in on the joke and began ordering bulk shipments so he could send them out as gifts.

David Life and Sharon Gannon continue to expand their business and yoga empire, with an increasing focus on social and environmental awareness. Their new flagship Manhattan studio has evolved into a "spiritual village," an enormous, full-service life and wellness center where you can take yoga classes, lounge in the café, browse in the bookstore, socialize with other yogis and, of course, shop.

Sandy and Bill McCauley are still teaching at their family-owned Yoga Loka studio in Sacramento. The branch in San Rafael where their daughter Vanessa taught has been sold. There's been no communication between Bikram and Yoga Loka since the settlement.

James Barkan is still teaching yoga and training new instructors at his studio in southern Florida. He continues to praise Bikram as his inspiration and mentor, although the two have not reconciled. "I think it would sort of be a moot point to reconcile. But I will always love Bikram. I will always consider him a family member, not just a friend," he says.

While nurturing dreams of opening his own place, Esak Garcia has been helping his friends open a Bikram studio in Lima, Peru. He continues to spread the gospel of competitive yoga, offering to help yogis prepare for the next Bikram Ghosh cup. He's had no luck landing an endorsement deal. So far.

In 2006 the Los Angeles city attorney charged Bikram Choudhury with ten criminal counts for failing to remedy safety violations at his Los Angeles studio, including overcrowding and failure to maintain adequate emergency exits. Bikram's company threatened to countersue for harassment but later pleaded no contest to three of the charges. Bikram subsequently announced plans to move his headquarters to Hawaii but hasn't yet done so.

Bikram was not able to convince Olympics organizers to include yoga at the 2008 Beijing Olympic Games. Nor has the International Olympic Committee given any indication that it's considering yoga for inclusion at the 2012 London games. That may *sound* like a no, but I wouldn't put money on it.

Yoga: A Rough and Spotty Chronology

Vedic Period (2000–1000 B.C.): The word *yoga* first appears in the Vedas, the sacred scriptures of Hinduism.

Pre-Classical Period (1000–500 B.C.): In the Upanishads, a set of Vedic hymns, yoga is defined as a discipline used to achieve liberation from suffering.

Classical Period (200 B.C.–A.D. 400): Patanjali (maybe) writes the Yoga Sutra, the first systematic presentation of yoga, and outlines an eight-limbed path aimed at eventual enlightenment.

Post-Classical Period (A.D. 400–A.D. 1900): Many yoga styles emerge, some based on elements of the Yoga Sutra. Around A.D. 1400 the Hatha Yoga Pradipika is written. Hatha yoga takes precedence.

1805: The Reverend William Emerson publishes the first translation of Sanskrit scripture in the United States.

1840s: His son, Ralph Waldo Emerson, takes an interest in the Bhagavad Gita and Eastern religion.

1875: Theosophical Society founded in New York.

1893: Charismatic guru Swami Vivekananda addresses the Parliament of the World's Religions in Chicago, and establishes the first Vedanta Society in New York City a year later.

1900–1924: The already large influx of South Asian immigrants to the West increases, particularly to the United States

1910: American yogi Pierre Bernard, "The Omnipotent Oom," is accused of abducting two young women.

1917: The Asiatic Barred Zone Act forbids immigration from Southeast Asia to the United States. Seven years later the United States places limits on Indian immigration; meanwhile, Americans begin traveling to India to study yoga.

1924: Tirumalai Krishnamacharya crosses paths with the maharaja of Mysore, and opens a yoga school in the Mysore Palace. Among his protégés are B.K.S. Iyengar, Pattabhi Jois, Indra Devi and T.K.V. Desikachar.

1930s: Cole Porter and Mae West are in the news for their interest in yoga.

1945: Theos Bernard, Pierre Bernard's nephew, publishes *Hatha Yoga: The Report of a Personal Experience*, one of the first guidebooks to yoga asanas.

1946: Swami Yogananda publishes *Autobiography of a Yogi.*

1947: After studying with yoga master Krishnamacharya in India, Indra Devi opens a yoga studio in Hollywood and attracts followers such as Elizabeth Arden and Greta Garbo.

1955: B.K.S. Iyengar first visits New York and teaches at the 92nd Street YMCA.

1960–1970: The postwar youth culture (the baby boomers) incorporate yoga. Yogananda's *Autobiography of a Yogi* gains readership in the United States with the post–World War Two generation.

1961: Richard Hittleman begins broadcasting the *Yoga for Health* TV program. Americans can now enjoy a decidedly unspiritual form of yoga via their televisions.

1965: The Asiatic Barred Zone Act is repealed. Indians can immigrate to America again. There is soon a wave of arriving gurus and spiritual leaders.

1965–1970: Ashrams and spiritual communities burgeon. Yoga is an integral part of their teachings.

1968: The Beatles study Transcendental Meditation with Maharishi Mahesh Yogi but soon fall out with him. Later John Lennon writes "Sexy Sadie" about his experience.

1969: Indian guru Swami Satchidananda opens the Woodstock Festival and teaches thousands of people to chant "om."

1970s: Westerners begin branding yoga asana "styles."

1970: Former Harvard professor and now-dropout Ram Dass tours college campuses with his book *Be Here Now.*

1975: First edition of *Yoga Journal,* the yoga industry's magazine of record, is published.

1980s: Yoga pervades the fitness industry.

1987: Iyengar Yoga Association of Greater New York is established.

1990: *Yoga Journal* notes a surge in attendance at yoga classes. Circulation has more than doubled in six years, to 70,000.

1993: *The Lancet,* an influential medical journal, publishes research indicating that lifestyle changes including yoga-based stress management can reverse heart disease.

1993: Jivamukti Yoga Center is established in New York City.

2003: First Bikram Yoga championships in the United States.

2005: *Yoga Journal*'s Yoga in America study concludes that yoga is a $3-billion-a-year business. In America alone 16.5 million people are practicing yoga.

2012: John Philp sweeps to victory in the Warrior Two Yoga Smackdown at the Baghdad Summer Olympics.
NB: The last one is a prediction.

NOTES

1. LIGHTS, KARMA, ACTION!

1. This and subsequent statements are taken from interviews with the author, Prescott, Arizona, 17 August 2004, and Chino Valley, Arizona, 29 August 2005.
2. This and subsequent statements are taken from an interview with the author, New York, 22 October 2004.
3. This and subsequent statements are taken from interviews with the author, Cumberland, Rhode Island, 13–15 September 2004.
4. This and subsequent statements are taken from interviews with the author, Fort Lauderdale, Florida, 26–27 October 2004 and 3 October 2005.
5. This and subsequent statements are taken from an interview with the author, New York, 20 October 2004.
6. This and subsequent statements are taken from interviews with the author, San Francisco, 13–14 October 2004.
7. This and subsequent statements are taken from an interview with the author, New York, 20 April 2005.

2. COWBOYS AND INDIANS

1. Richard G. Geldard and Robert Richardson, *The Spiritual Teachings of Ralph Waldo Emerson,* 2nd ed. (Great Barrington, MA: Lindisfarne Books, 2001), 55.
2. This and subsequent statements are taken from an interview with the author, New York, 20 April 2005.
3. "Swami Vivekananda at the Parliament of Religions," Vedanta Center of Atlanta, www.vedanta-atlanta.org/articles/vivekananda/parliament. html (accessed 1 June 2008).
4. "Hindus at the Fair," *Boston Evening Transcript,* 30 September 1893.
5. "South Asian Pioneers in California, 1899–1965," chap. 4 of *Echoes of Freedom: South Asian Pioneers in California, 1899–1965,* The Library, University of California, Berkeley, http://www.lib.berkeley.edu/ SSEAL/echoes/chapter4/chapter4.html (accessed 12 November 2007).
6. Hugh B. Urban, *Tantra: Sex, Secrecy, Politics, and Power in the Study of Religion* (Berkeley: University of California Press, 2003), 209.

7. Robert Love, "Fear of Yoga," *Columbia Journalism Review,* November/December 2006, http://cjrarchives.org/issues/2006/6/love.asp (accessed 7 November 2007).

8. Ibid.

9. Ibid.

10. Ibid.

11. "Guru's Exit," *Time,* 4 August 1952, http://www.time.com/time/magazine/article/0,9171,822420,00.html (accessed 13 November 2007).

12. Love, "Fear of Yoga."

13. Aleister Crowley, "Eight Lectures on Yoga," http://deoxy.org/annex/Eight_Lectures_on_Yoga.pdf (accessed 22 November 2007).

14. Indra Devi, "Yoga for You," World Vegetarian Congress, http://www.ivu.org/congress/wvc57/souvenir/devi.html (accessed 12 January 2008).

15. Adriana Aboy, "Indra Devi's Legacy," *Hinduism Today,* October–December 2002, http://www.hinduismtoday.com/archives/2002/10-12/52-54_indradevi.shtml (accessed 28 November 2007).

3. POSERS

1. Andrea Ferretti, "Yogi Baron," www.yogajournal.com, http://www.yogajournal.com/lifestyle/1935 (accessed 1 August 2008).

2. "The Cost of Incarceration," *Time,* 16 September 1966, http://www.time.com/time/magazine/article/0,9171,836373-1,00.html (accessed 12 December 2007).

3. Ray Connolly, "Is It Arise Sir Ringo?" *Daily Mail,* 22 December 2006, http://www.dailymail.co.uk/tvshowbiz/article-424456/Is-arise-Sir-Ringo.html (accessed 29 October 2008).

4. Dmitry Murashev, "John Lennon and Paul McCartney Interview for NBC program 'The Tonight Show' (1968, May 14)," DM's Beatles Site, http://www.dmbeatles.com/interviews.php?interview=64 (accessed 30 November, 2007).

5. "When Maharishi Threw Beatles Out," *Times of India,* 15 February 2006, http://timesofindia.indiatimes.com/India/When_Maharishi_threw_Beatles_out/articleshow/msid-1415230,curpg-1.cms (accessed 11 December 2007).

6. John Lennon, Yoko Ono, David Sheff and G. Barry Golson, *All We Are Saying: The Last Major Interview with John Lennon and Yoko Ono* (New York: Macmillan, 2000), 191.

7. John Lennon, *Rolling Stone,* 7 January 1971, 39, cited by Jann Wenner in *Lennon Remembers* (London: Verso, 2001), 52.

8. This and subsequent statements are taken from an interview with the author, Berkeley, California, 12 October 2004.

9. Richard Corliss, "The New Ideal of Beauty," *Time,* 30 August 1982, http://www.time.com/time/magazine/article/0,9171,921278-5,00. html (accessed 4 January 2008).

10. Aljean Harmetz, "Hollywood: This Way In," *New York Times,* 13 March 1983, http://query.nytimes.com/gst/fullpage.html?res= 9A03E1DB1539F930A25750C0A965948260&sec=travel&spon=&p agewanted=2 (accessed 30 October 2008).

11. "Losing Weight and Keeping It Off," CNN.com, 13 October 2002, http://transcripts.cnn.com/TRANSCRIPTS/0210/13/sm.06.html (accessed 5 January 2008).

12. Joel Kramer and Diana Alstad, "On Yoga and Evolution," White Lotus Foundation, http://www.whitelotus.org/library2/articles/kramer_ alstad/evolution/index.shtml (accessed 5 January 2008).

13. Otto Friedrich, "New Age Harmonies," *Time,* 7 December 1987, http://www.time.com/time/magazine/article/0,9171,966129- 11,00.html (accessed 8 January 2008).

14. Martha Smilgis, Mary Cronin and Michael Riley, "A New Age Dawning," *Time,* 31 August 1987, http://aolsvc.timeforkids.kol.aol. com/time/magazine/article/0,9171,965314,00.html (accessed 8 January 2008).

15. See "Can Lifestyle Changes Reverse Coronary Heart Disease?" National Center for Biotechnology Information, http://www.ncbi. nlm.nih.gov/pubmed/1973470?dopt=Abstract (accessed 8 January 2008).

16. Holly Hammond, "Meet the Innovators/Dean Ornish, M.D.," yoga-journal.com, http://www.yogajournal.com/lifestyle/359 (accessed 8 January 2008).

17. Barbara Whitaker, "Now in the H.M.O.: Yoga Teachers and Naturopaths," *New York Times,* 24 November 1996, http://query. nytimes.com/gst/fullpage.html?res=9501E6DC143DF937A15752C1 A960958260&sec=health&spon=&pagewanted=all (accessed 12 January 2008).

18. Jane E. Brody, "Relaxation Method May Aid Health," *New York Times,* 7 August 1996, http://query.nytimes.com/gst/fullpage.html?res=

9B0CE7D7163EF934A3575BC0A960958260 (accessed 12 January 2008).

19. Anne Cushman, "Power Yoga," *Yoga Journal,* January/February 1995, http://www.natural-connection.com/resource/yoga_journal/power_yoga.html (accessed 12 January 2008).

20. Ann Powers, "Pop View: New Tune for the Material Girl I'm Neither," *New York Times,* 1 March 1998, http://query.nytimes.com/gst/fullpage.html?res=9D07E0DB153EF932A35750C0A96E958260 (accessed 12 January 2008).

21. Lygia Barnett, "Madonna's Reinvention," *Women's Fitness and Health,* http://www.dannyparadise.com/pdf/madonna1.pdf (accessed 12 January 2008).

22. This and subsequent statements are taken from an interview with the author, New York, 8 December 2004.

23. This and subsequent statements are taken from an interview with the author, New York, 22 October 2004.

24. "Yoga Party," Entertainment Weekly Online, 13 March 1998, http://www.ew.com/ew/article/0,,282173,00.html (accessed 22 January 2008).

25. "Celebrity Central: Madonna," People Online, http://www.people.com/people/madonna (accessed 22 January 2008).

26. This and subsequent statements are taken from an interview with the author, San Jose, California, 13 October 2004.

27. Dayna Macy, "Yoga Journal Releases 2008 'Yoga in America' Market Study," yogajournal.com, http://www.yogajournal.com/advertise/press_releases/10 (accessed 22 January 2008).

28. "Press, Statistics, Resources and Links," North American Studio Alliance, http://www.namasta.com/pressresources.php#7 (accessed 22 January 2008).

29. "World Yoga Survey," YogaSurvey.com, http://www.yogainaustralia.com/ (accessed 22 January 2008).

30. Nicole Brydson, "Manhattan Yoga Mania: Celebrity Mat Spreads as Jivamukti Opens," *New York Observer,* 28 May 2006, http://www.observer.com/node/38922 (accessed 30 January 2008).

31. All dollar amounts are in U.S. dollars unless otherwise specified.

32. Becky Barrow, "'Spiritual Spending' Costs Women £670m a Year," Telegraph Online, 8 October 2003, http://www.telegraph.co.uk/news/uknews/1443571/Spiritual-spending-costs-women-£670m-a-year.html (accessed 30 January 2008).

33. This and subsequent statements are taken from interviews with the author, Rhinebeck, New York, 13 June 2004, and New York City, 22 October 2004.

34. Mary Billard, "Flow or No, Following the Yogis," *New York Times,* 18 February 2005, http://travel.nytimes.com/2005/02/18/travel/escapes/18yoga.html?scp=2&sq=%22Yoga+Journal%22&st=nyt (accessed 14 February 2008).

35. Erica Rodefer, "Retreat Yourself," yogajournal.com, http://www.yogajournal.com/lifestyle/2316?page=1 (accessed 14 February 2008).

36. "Omega's History: A Pioneer in Holistic Studies and the Personal Growth Retreat," http://www.eomega.org/omega/about/history/ (accessed 8 October 2007).

37. This and subsequent statements are taken from an interview with the author, New York, 22 October 2004.

38. Brian Morrissey, "Lexus Is Back with Usual Christmas Downer," Adfreak.com, 27 November 2007, http://adweek.blogs.com/adfreak/2007/11/bmw-lexus-merry.html (accessed 21 October 2007).

4. McYOGA

1. "Change Peoples' Lives & Earn a Great Living Teaching Yoga…," Sonic Yoga Center for Yoga Studies, http://www.sonicyoga.com/2006/teach.htm (accessed 9 October 2007).

2. This and subsequent statements from Wrubel and Lichter are taken from interviews with the author, New York, 3 May 2005.

3. "Directors: Ganga White," White Lotus Foundation, http://www.whitelotus.org/directors/ganga/index.shtml (accessed 22 October 2007).

4. Maria Hummel, "Everything's Not Zen," *LA Weekly,* 4 November 2004, http://www.laweekly.com/news/features/everythings-not-zen/1221/?page=1 (accessed 22 October 2007).

5. Ibid.

6. *Sunstone assures potential franchisees:* "The Sunstone Advantage," http://www.sunstoneyoga.com/FranchiseInformation/TheSunstoneAdvantage/tabid/283/Default.aspx (October 5, 2008); *To properly outfit a studio:* "Sunstone Yoga," http://yoga.lovetoknow.com/Sunstone_Yoga (accessed 5 October 2008); *Some estimates go as high:* Valerie McTavish, "Downward Dog Eat Dog," *BC Business,* 1 February 2008, http://www.bcbusinessonline.ca/bcb/top-stories/2008/02/01/downward-dog-eat-dog (accessed 5 October 2008).

7. Hilary E. Macgregor, "Assuming the Profit Position," *Los Angeles Times,* 10 September 2004, http://articles.latimes.com/2004/sep/10/health/he-yogaworks10 (accessed 11 November 2007).

8. This and subsequent statements are taken from an interview with the author, New York, 7 May 2005.

9. This and subsequent statements are taken from an interview with the author, New York, 1 October 2004.

10. This and subsequent statements are taken from an interview with the author, New York, 6 October 2004.

5. THE GURU WHO LAID THE GOLDEN EGG

1. "Bikram Choudhury," I Love India, http://www.iloveindia.com/spirituality/gurus/bikram-choudhary.html (accessed 5 December 2007).

2. "Nixon: Surgery, Shock and Uncertainty," *Time,* 11 November 1974, http://www.time.com/time/magazine/article/0,9171,911480,00.html (accessed 12 December 2007).

3. "'Hot' Yoga Burns Bright," *CBS 60 Minutes,* 8 June 2005, http://www.bikramyoga.com/CBS60Minutes.htm (accessed 14 December 2007).

4. Robert Garcia, "Re: Interview Request," 28 July 2004, personal email.

5. This and subsequent statements are taken from interviews with the author, San Francisco, 15 October 2004, Chicago, 26–31 July 2005, and New York, 10 November 2005.

6. Hilary E. Macgregor, "Had Your McYoga Today? A Stretch of Success," *Los Angeles Times,* 7 July 2002, http://articles.latimes.com/2002/jul/07/news/lv-bikram7 (accessed 16 December 2007).

7. Neil Chatterjee and Sophie Hardach, "Hollywood Guru Bikram Sells Yoga to 'Ugly Society,'" Reuters India, 3 March 2008, http://in.reuters.com/article/lifestyleMolt/idINSYD24390620080303 (accessed 16 December 2007).

8. Ibid.

9. This and subsequent statements are taken from an interview with the author's film crew, Los Angeles, 20 February 2005.

10. This and subsequent statements are taken from an interview with the author, San Rafael, California, 25 March 2004.

11. Ibid.

12. Julian Guthrie, "McYoga for the Masses: Popular Yogi to Franchise Ancient Indian Discipline," *San Francisco Chronicle,* 10 November 2002, http://www.sfgate.com/cgi-bin/article.cgi?file=/c/a/2002/11/10/MN194695.DTL (accessed 27 June 2008).

13. Ibid.
14. "Bikram Yoga Teacher Training Faq's," Bikramyoga.com, http://www.bikramyoga.com/TeacherTraining/ttfaqs.htm (accessed 29 June 2008).
15. "Monk Gloats over Yoga Championship," *The Onion* 29 (8), http://dananau.com/wabe/humor/monkgloats.pdf (accessed 26 November 2007).
16. Interview with the author, Los Angeles, 27 September 2003.
17. Film footage of yogis on stage performing poses for the film *Yoga, Inc.*, Bad Dog Tales, Inc., 2007. It's unclear whether the footage is of a competition.
18. Interview with the author, Los Angeles, 28 September 2003.
19. Interview with the author, New York, 23 October 2004.

6. KARMA POLICE

1. This and subsequent statements are taken from an interview with the author, New York, 20 April 2005.
2. Jennifer Barrett, "Ethical Dilemma," *Yoga Journal,* March/April 2004, http://www.yjevents.com/views/1211_1.cfm (accessed 21 March 2008).
3. "Yoga Alliance Code of Conduct," Yoga Alliance, http://www.yogaalliance.org/Conduct.html (accessed 21 March 2008).
4. "Code of Professional Standards," California Yoga Teachers Association, http://www.yogateachersassoc.org/ethics/ (accessed 21 March 2008).
5. "Application Form, 200-Hour Certification in the Kripalu Tradition," Discovery Yoga, http://www.discoveryyoga.com/YTT.htm#YTT200 (accessed 21 March 2008).
6. "Code of Professional Standards for Kundalini Yoga Teachers," Yoga House, http://www.yogahouse.org/PDFs/Ethics_Conduct.pdf (accessed 21 March 2008).
7. "Code of Ethics," Iyengar Yoga Association of Canada, http://iyengaryogacanada.com/teachers_codeofethics.php (accessed 21 March 2008).
8. "Ethics, Equity & Welfare," The British Wheel of Yoga, http://www.bwy.org.uk/about/ethics.php (accessed 21 March 2008).
9. "IYTA Code of Ethics," International Yoga Teachers Association of Australia, http://www.iyta.org.au/ethics.html (accessed 26 March 2008).

10. "Yogalicious!" *People*, 9 June 2003, http://www.baronbaptiste.com/pages/people2.htm (accessed 21 March 2008).

11. Jeff Wagenheim, "Gods and Monsters," *Yoga Journal*, September/October 1999, http://www.yjevents.com/views/288_1.cfm (accessed 11 April 2008).

12. "B.C. School Yoga Classes Slammed," CBC News, 9 January 2007, http://www.cbc.ca/canada/british-columbia/story/2007/01/09/bc-yoga.html?ref=rss (accessed 11 April 2008).

13. Holly Vicente Robaina, "The Truth about Yoga," *Today's Christian Woman*, March/April 2005, 40, http://www.christianitytoday.com/tcw/2005/marapr/14.40.html?start=2 (accessed 24 April 2008).

14. Lisa Takeuchi Cullen, Mahtomedi, "Stretching for Jesus," *Time*, 29 August 2005, http://www.time.com/time/magazine/article/0,9171,1098937,00.html (accessed 24 April 2008).

15. Sam O'Neal, "Yoga Is a Stretch," *Leadership Journal*, Spring 2007, http://www.christianitytoday.com/le/2007/002/15.11.html (accessed 24 April 2008).

16. Congregation for the Doctrine of the Faith, "Letter to the Bishops of the Catholic Church on Some Aspects of Christian Meditation," 15 October 1989, http://www.cin.org/users/james/files/meditation.htm (accessed 28 October 2008); Timothy Shriver, "Yoga Challenge for the Pope," *Washington Post*, 7 April 2008, http://newsweek.washington-post.com/onfaith/religionfromtheheart/2008/04/benedict_xvis_upcoming_visit_t.html (accessed 29 October 2008).

7. CHASING A YOGA BUTT

1. Ibid.

2. See Susi Hately Aldous, "Anatomy and Asana: Preventing Yoga Injuries," http://www.anatomyandasana.com/workshops.htm (accessed 29 April 2008).

3. This and subsequent statements are taken from interviews with the author, New York, 3 November 2004 and 8 December 2004.

4. Lorraine Kreahling, "When Does Flexible Become Harmful? 'Hot' Yoga Draws Fire," *New York Times*, 30 March 2004, http://query.nytimes.com/gst/fullpage.html?res=9905EFDE1F30F933A05750C0A9629C8B63 (accessed 30 April 2008).

5. This and subsequent statements are taken from a series of interviews with the author, New York, November–December 2004.

6. Nora Isaacs, "The Yoga Therapist Will See You Now," *New York Times,* 10 May 2007, http://www.nytimes.com/2007/05/10/fashion/10Fitness.html (accessed 30 April 2008).

7. "Yoga-Based Cancer Rehabilitation Program," ClinicalTrials.gov, September 2005, http://clinicaltrials.gov/ct2/show/NCT00179348 (accessed 30 April 2008).

8. "Clinical Trials," The Johns Hopkins Arthritis Center, http://www.hopkins-arthritis.org/arthritis-research/clin_trials.html (accessed 9 May 2008).

9. Rachel Shabi, "Omming on Empty," *The Guardian,* 26 February 2005, http://www.guardian.co.uk/weekend/story/0,3605,1425223,00.html (accessed 9 May 2008).

10. Devon Haynie, "Yoga: A New Way to Fight Anorexia and Bulimia," Columbia News Service, 13 February 2007, http://jscms.jrn.columbia.edu/cns/2007-02-13/haynie-yogatherapy (accessed 9 May 2008).

11. Lynn Ginsburg and Mary Taylor, *What Are You Hungry For? Women, Food, and Spirituality* (New York: St. Martin's Press, 2002), http://www.whatareyouhungryfor.net/ (accessed 9 May 2008).

12. "Yoga and Anorexia," Yoga.com: Forums, http://www.yoga.com/forums/forums/thread-view.asp?tid=15973&posts=9 (accessed 9 May 2008).

13. This and subsequent statements are taken from an interview with the author, New York, 12 August 2004.

14. Pamela Paul, "When Yoga Hurts," *Time,* 4 October 2007, http://www.time.com/time/magazine/article/0,9171,1668470,00.html (accessed 9 May 2008).

15. This and subsequent statements are taken from an interview with the author, New York, 12 August 2004.

16. Lisa Maria, "Yoga's Silent Scandal," *Whole Life Times,* April 2006, http://wholelifetimes.com/2006/04/yogasex0604.html (accessed 9 May 2008).

17. Paul Keegan, "Yogis Behaving Badly," *Business 2.0,* September 2002, http://www.rickross.com/reference/general/general478.html (accessed 9 May 2008).

18. David Frawley, "Yoga, Ahimsa and the Terrorist Attacks," *The Hindu,* 13 November 2001, http://www.hinduonnet.com/thehindu/op/2001/11/13/stories/2001111300050100.htm (accessed 9 May 2008).

8. STRETCHING THE SATYA

1. Eknath Easwaran, *Gandhi, the Man: The Story of His Transformation* (Tomales, CA: Nilgiri Press, 1997), 151.

2. Dennis Dalton, *Mahatma Gandhi: Nonviolent Power in Action* (New York: Columbia University Press, 2001), 12.

3. B.N. Ghosh, *Gandhian Political Economy: Principles, Practice and Policy* (Aldershot, UK: Ashgate Publishing, 2007), 62.

4. Sri Aurobindo, *India's Rebirth: A Selection from Sri Aurobindo's Writings, Talks and Speeches* (Paris: Institut de Recherches Evolutives, 2000), http://www.voi.org/books/ir/IR_part3.htm (accessed 23 May 2008).

5. David J. Craig, "Current Indian and Pakistani Tensions Subject of Address by Gandhi's Grandson," B.U. Bridge, 29 October 1999, http://www.bu.edu/bridge/archive/1999/10-29/features3.html (accessed 23 May 2008).

6. This and subsequent statements are taken from an interview with the author, Princeton, Massachusetts, 16 September 2004.

7. "Yoga versus Pilates," *elements living,* 7 July 2004, http://magazine. elementsliving.tv/index.php?option=com_content&task=view&id=6 &Itemid=1 (accessed 23 May 2008).

8. "Face-Off: Striking a Pose," *Folio,* 1 November 2003, http:// findarticles.com/p/articles/mi_m3065/is_11_32/ai_109384465/ pg_1 (accessed 23 May 2008).

9. "Face-Off," *Folio.*

10. Swami Nirmalananda Giri, "The Foundations of Yoga," Atma Jyoti Ashram, http://www.atmajyoti.org/med_foundations_of_yoga.asp (accessed 26 May 2008).

11. Sarah Bowen Shea, "The Better Sex Workout," *Women's Health,* 30 November 2007, http://www.womenshealthmag.com/fitness/the-sex-benefits-of-yoga (accessed 30 May 2008).

12. "Yoga Guru Accepts Doctors' Challenge to Cure Cancer Patient," India eNews, 7 January 2008, http://www.indiaenews.com/health/ 20080107/90135.htm (accessed 4 June 2008).

13. "What Cult Were You In," Cult Education Forum, http://forum. rickross.com/read.php?5,151,page=1 (accessed 4 June 2008).

14. "Shaja Yoga," Cult Education Forum, http://forum.rickross.com/ read.php?5,9316 (accessed 4 June 2008).

15. "Testimonials—Self Realization through Sahaja Yoga," Sahaja Yoga, http://www.sahajayoga.org/testimonials/default.asp (accessed 4 June 2008).

16. "So Just What Is This Cool Breeze?" http://www.geocities.com/breezeofspirit/personal.htm (accessed 4 June 2008).

17. "Interview with Shri Mataji," *Sahaja Yoga Meditation: Talks,* 1 August 2003, http://www.irelandyoga.org/talks/voa-itv-interview-with-shri-mataji-182003/interview-with-shri-mataji-pg-14/ (accessed 9 June 2008).

18. "About ISY RHC," *The International Sahaja Yoga Research and Health Centre,* http://www.sahajahealthcentre.com/about_sy_rhc.htm (accessed 9 June 2008).

19. Paul Keegan, "Yogis Behaving Badly," *Business 2.0,* September 2002, http://www.rickross.com/reference/general/general478.html (accessed 12 June 2008).

20. Interview with the author, Princeton, Massachusetts, 1 August 2004.

21. "Bikram Yoga: Testimonials," Bikram's Yoga College of India, http://www.bikramyoga.com/Testimonials.html (accessed 14 August 2008).

22. "Bikram Yoga: The Benefits," Bikram's Yoga College of India, http://www.bikramyoga.com/Yoga/Benefits.htm (accessed 14 August 2008).

23. Dr. Joel Brame, "Five Ways to Reverse Cancer Using Bikram Yoga," http://www.joelbrame.com/uploads/Dr._Brame_-_Can_Bikram_Yoga_Reverse_Cancer_Processes.pdf (accessed 14 August 2008).

24. Swami Chidananda, "Yoga: What It Is and What It Is Not," Yoga-Age.com, http://www.yoga-age.com/articles/chida1.html (accessed 11 July 2008).

25. Professor Seshagiri Rao, "Yoga and Ecumenism: An Interview with Georg Feuerstein," Traditional Yoga Studies, 2007, http://www.traditionalyogastudies.com/articles_miscellaneous_ecumenism.html (accessed 11 July 2008).

26. "Yoga-Based Intervention for Carpal Tunnel Syndrome," *Journal of the American Medical Association* 280 (18): 1601–03, http://jama.ama-assn.org/cgi/content/abstract/280/18/1601 (accessed 11 July 2008).

27. "Comparing Yoga, Exercise, and a Self-Care Book for Chronic Low Back Pain," *Annals of Internal Medicine* 143 (12): 849–56, http://www.annals.org/cgi/content/full/143/12/849 (accessed 11 July 2008).

28. See "Yoga for Asthma," Natural Ways to Health, http://www.naturalways.com/yoga-asthma.htm (accessed 11 July 2008).

29. S. Cooper, J. Oborne, S. Newton, V. Harrison, C. Thompson, S. Lewis and A. Tattersfield, "Effect of Two Breathing Exercises (Buteyko and Pranayama) in Asthma: A Randomised Controlled Trial," *Thorax* 58 (8): 674–79, http://www.pubmedcentral.nih.gov/articlerender.fcgi? artid=1746772 (accessed 11 July 2008).

30. G.B. Marks, "Sahaja Yoga in the Management of Moderate to Severe Asthma: A Randomised Controlled Trial," *Thorax* 57: 110–15, http://thorax.bmj.com/cgi/content/abstract/57/2/110 (accessed 11 July 2008).

31. Kate Stinchfield, "Skip the Botox: Try Facial Yoga," *Time,* 13 November 2007, http://www.time.com/time/health/article/0,8599, 1683386,00.html (accessed 11 July 2008).

32. Aja Mangum, "Downward Drooping Cheeks," *New York,* 4 February 2008, http://nymag.com/beauty/features/43568/ (accessed 11 July 2008).

33. "lululemon manifesto," lululemon athletica, http://www.lululemon. com/culture/manifesto (accessed 11 July 2008).

34. Louise Story, " 'Seaweed' Clothing Has None, Tests Show," *New York Times,* 14 November 2007, http://www.nytimes.com/2007/11/14/ business/14seaweed.html?pagewanted=1&_r=2&ei=5088&en=0bcc8 3e54552c597&ex=1352696400&partner=rssnyt&emc=rss (accessed 11 July 2008).

35. Eileen Delehanty Pearkes, "Seaweed Yoga," *Ascent,* 19 November 2007, http://ascentmagazine.net/wordpress/?p=173 (accessed 21 July 2008).

36. Tara, "Is There, or Isn't There, Seaweed in lululemon Clothes?" yoga-journal.com, 19 November 2007, http://blogs.yogajournal.com/ yogabuzz/2007/11/is_there_or_isnt_there_seaweed.html#comments (accessed 21 July 2008).

37. "Bad lululemon Experience," discovervancouver.com, http://www. discovervancouver.com/forum/bad-lululemon-experience-t43073.html&st=150 (accessed 21 November 2008).

38. Peter Foster, "Lululemon Asked for It," *Financial Post,* 16 November 2007, http://www.financialpost.com/story.html?id=589fb9e5-c143-48f4-99b7-7171630e8546&k=43929&p=2 (accessed 21 November 2008).

39. "lululemon Drops Coke and Pepsi from Its Manifesto," Canadian Press, 16 January 2008, http://www.marketingmag.ca/english/news/ marketer/article.jsp?content=20080116_777333_2090 (accessed 21 November 2008).

40. "Frequently Asked Questions and Answers," lululemon athletica, http://www.lululemon.com/about/faq (accessed 21 November 2008).

41. Jane Brody, "Reports of Psychosis after Erhard Course: Doctors Tell of 7 Who Developed Severe Disturbance after Taking Self-Awareness Seminars," *New York Times,* 24 April 1977, http://select.nytimes.com/gst/abstract.html?res=F60616FC395812718DDDAD0A94DC405B878BF1D3&scp=2&sq=%22erhard%22&st=p&oref=login (accessed 21 November 2008).

42. "Notices: The Landmark Forum; Landmark Education Transfer & Cancellation Policy," Landmark Education, http://www.landmarkeducation.com/display_content.jsp?top=24&mid=343610 (accessed 11 December 2008).

43. Bruce Constantineau, "Profits Soar at Lululemon," *Vancouver Sun,* 2 April 2008, http://www.canada.com/vancouversun/news/business/story.html?id=7d4a6589-01e7-4d07-bb24-5b324eb651e4&k=62474 (accessed 11 December 2008).

44. Rick Aristotle Munarriz, "Turning lululemon into Lemonade," *Vancouver Sun,* 2 April 2008, http://www.fool.com/investing/general/2008/04/02/turning-lululemon-into-lemonade.aspx (accessed 11 December 2008).

9. STEAL THIS YOGA

1. This and subsequent statements from Bill McCauley, Sandy McCauley and Vanessa Calder are taken from an interview with the author, San Rafael, California, 25 March 2004.

2. Julian Guthrie, "McYoga for the Masses: Popular Yogi to Franchise Ancient Indian Discipline," *San Francisco Chronicle,* 10 November 2002, http://www.sfgate.com/cgi-bin/article.cgi?file=/c/a/2002/11/10/MN194695.DTL (accessed 14 July 2008).

3. This and subsequent statements are taken from an interview with the author, New York, 2 May 2004.

4. Joshua Kurlantzick, "The Money Pose," *Mother Jones,* March/April 2005, http://www.motherjones.com/news/dispatch/2005/03/Money_Pose.html (accessed 14 July 2008).

5. This and subsequent statements are taken from an interview with the author, San Francisco, 20 June 2005.

6. "Our Mission," Open Source Yoga Unity, http://www.yogaunity.org/ (accessed 14 July 2008).

7. Vanessa Grigoriadis, "Controlled Breathing, in the Extreme," *New York Times,* 6 July 2003, http://query.nytimes.com/gst/fullpage.html?res=9B01E3D61E3AF935A35754C0A9659C8B63&sec=&spon=&pagewanted=2 (accessed 14 July 2008).

8. This and subsequent statements are taken from an interview with the author, Berkeley, California, 26 March 2004.

9. John Heilemann, "The Choirboy," *New York,* 21 May 2005, http://nymag.com/nymetro/news/features/12061/ (accessed 14 July 2008).

10. "Jivamukti® Yoga Teacher Training: 300-Hour Residential Program," Omega Institute, http://eomega.org/pdfs/SM08-0626-249.pdf (accessed 14 July 2008).

11. James Greenberg, "Asana™," *Yoga Journal,* December 2003, http://www.yjevents.com/views/1143_1.cfm (accessed 12 August 2008).

12. Paul Keegan, "Yogis Behaving Badly," *Business 2.0,* September 2002, http://www.rickross.com/reference/general/general478.html (accessed 12 August 2008).

13. "Sweaty Studio Sessions," September 2007, http://sweatystudiosessions.blogspot.com/2007/09/bikram-yoga-union-square-new-york-city.html (accessed 2 August 2008).

14. Laura Fraser, "Bouncing into Graceland," yogajournal.com, http://www.yogajournal.com/lifestyle/1331 (accessed 8 August 2008).

15. Suketu Mehta, "A Big Stretch," *New York Times,* 7 May 2007, http://www.nytimes.com/2007/05/07/opinion/07mehta.html (accessed 8 August 2008).

16. Siddharth Srivastava, "It's Patently Obvious," *Asia Times,* 2 July 2005, http://www.atimes.com/atimes/South_Asia/GG02Df02.html (accessed 5 August 2008).

17. Kama Sutra: Making Love Better, http://www.kamasutra.com (accessed 12 June 2008).

18. Suketu Mehta, "A Big Stretch," *New York Times,* 7 May 2007, http://www.nytimes.com/2007/05/07/opinion/07mehta.html (accessed 8 August 2008).

10. OM FOR WAYWARD BOYS

1. "About the Ashram," Shree Muktananda Ashram, http://www.siddhayoga.org/shree-muktananda-ashram (accessed 21 June 2008).

2. Associated Press, "Hindus Upset over Myers' 'Love Guru,'" msnbc.com, 28 March 2008, http://www.msnbc.msn.com/id/23834381/ (accessed 21 June 2008).

3. Anne Simpkinson, "Soul Betrayal," Common Boundary Inc., November/December 1996, http://www.advocateweb.org/HOPE/ soulbetrayal.asp (accessed 23 June 2008).

4. "Kripalu," *Hinduism Today,* September 1989, http://www.hinduism today.com/archives/1989/09/1989-09-02.shtml (accessed 23 June 2008).

5. "History of Kripalu Center," Kripalu Center for Yoga and Health, http://www.kripalu.org/about_us/491 (accessed 23 June 2008).

6. Claudia Cummins, "Life without Sex," *Yoga Journal,* November 2002, http://www.yjevents.com/views/770_1.cfm (accessed 23 June 2008).

7. This and subsequent statements are taken from an interview with the author, New York, 20 April 2005.

8. Geoffrey D. Falk, *Stripping the Gurus: Sex, Violence, Abuse and Enlightenment* (Toronto: Million Monkeys Press, 2007), 128, http://www.strippingthegurus.com/stgsamplechapters/muktananda.asp (accessed 23 June 2008).

9. "Leaving Siddha Yoga," http://www.leavingsiddhayoga.net/ leaving.htm (accessed 23 June 2008).

10. "Instant Energy," *Time,* 26 July 1976, http://www.time.com/time/ magazine/article/0,9171,914413-1,00.html (accessed 23 June 2008).

11. Mark Healy, "Havens: The 'Bhajan Belt'; Serenity in the Catskills," *New York Times,* 18 October 2002, http://query.nytimes.com/gst/ fullpage.html?res=9902E6DF123DF93BA25753C1A9649C8B63&se c=&pagewanted=all (accessed 28 June 2008).

12. "Instant Energy," *Time,* 26 July 1976, http://www.time.com/time/ magazine/article/0,9171,914413-1,00.html (accessed 23 June 2008).

13. Lis Harris, "O Guru, Guru, Guru," *New Yorker,* 14 November 1994, 92, http://www.ex-cult.org/Groups/SYDA-Yoga/leave.txt (accessed 25 June 2008).

14. William Rodarmor, "The Secret Life of Swami Muktananda," *CoEvolution Quarterly,* 1983, http://www.ex-cult.org/Groups/ SYDA-Yoga/leave.txt (accessed 25 June 2008).

15. Stan Trout (Swami Abhayananda), "An Open Letter of Resignation from Swami Abhayananda to Muktananda," September 1981, http://www.ex-cult.org/Groups/SYDA-Yoga/syda.3 (accessed 25 June 2008).

16. Some People Who Have Left Siddha Yoga, "An Open Letter about Siddha Yoga," http://www.ex-cult.org/Groups/SYDA-Yoga/syda.2 (accessed 25 June 2008).

17. Each of these sites discusses the idea of GM and Afif as "lovers," though none offers proof: http://www.caic.org.au/eastern/sydda/syda1.htm, http://www.leavingsiddhayoga.net/ifeel.htm, http://www.ex-cult.org/Groups/SYDA-Yoga/aol-syda-discussion-1http://www.ex-cult.org/Groups/SYDA-Yoga/aol-syda-discussion-1, http://www.ex-cult.org/Groups/SYDA-Yoga/aol-syda-discussion-2, http://guruphiliac.blogspot.com/2006/07/mystery-of-missing-devi.html.

18. Matthew Cheng Sr., Ph.D., "Integral Yoga Institute—Yogaville: A Father's Story," Free Catherine, July 1999, http://www.freecatherine.com (accessed 25 June 2008).

19. Heather Yakin, "Yoga Group, Homeowners Target Project in Fallsburg," *Times Herald-Record,* 17 March 2006, http://archive.recordonline.com/archive/2006/03/17/news-hysuit-03-17.html (accessed 11 July 2008).

20. Matt Youngfrau, "SYDA Staying, but in Reduced Form," *Sullivan County Democrat,* 29 November 2002, http://161.58.174.199/archives/2002/news/11November/29/syda.html (accessed 11 July 2008).

21. Barbara McMahon, "Meg Ryan Isn't Giving Up Her Guru for Anyone," *Sunday Herald,* 30 July 2000, http://findarticles.com/p/articles/mi_qn4156/is_20000730/ai_n13952573 (accessed 11 July 2008).

22. Philip Self, "An Interview with John Friend," Anusara Yoga® in the Community, http://www.anusara.com/?pagerequested=article&article_id=27 (accessed 11 July 2008).

23. Elizabeth Gilbert, *Eat, Pray, Love* (New York: Penguin, 2007), 124, 127.

24. Richard K. Rein, "The Daughter of Jonestown Victim Leo Ryan Argues That Her Guru's Sect Is Not a Cult," *People,* 16 February 1981, http://www.people.com/people/archive/article/0,,20078618,00.html (accessed 21 July 2008).

25. Ben Fong-Torres, "Harrison Had Love-Haight Relationship with S.F." *San Francisco Chronicle,* 2 December 2001, http://www.sfgate.com/cgi-bin/article.cgi?f=/chronicle/archive/2001/12/02/MN235869.DTL&type=news (accessed 5 August 2008).

26. Victoria Moran, "Yoga Couples: Donna Fone and Rodney Yee," *Yoga Journal,* January/February 2001, http://www.yjevents.com/views/306_1.cfm (accessed 7 August 2008).

27. Charlie Goodyear and Rona Marech, "Yoga Guru in Compromising Position," *San Francisco Chronicle*, 12 May 2002, http://www.sfgate.com/cgi-bin/article.cgi?file=/chronicle/archive/2002/05/12/MN14618.DTL (accessed 7 August 2008).

28. Richard Corliss, "The Power of Yoga," *Time*, 15 April 2001, http://www.time.com/time/health/article/0,8599,106356,00.html (accessed 7 August 2008).

29. Goodyear and Marech, "Yoga Guru in Compromising Position."

30. Louise Danielle Palmer, "SELF Report: Compromising Positions," *SELF*, April 2004, http://www.self.com/magazine/articles/2006/05/15/0404yoga_single_page (accessed 7 August 2008).

31. Constance Loizos, "Yoga Stretches Far, from India to San Francisco," *San Francisco Chronicle*, 18 January 2004, E-1, http://www.sfgate.com/cgi-bin/article.cgi?f=/c/a/2004/01/18/LVGJM48H3F1.DTL (accessed 10 August 2008).

32. Abigail Pogrebin, "An Illicit Yoga Love Story," *New York*, 21 May 2005, http://nymag.com/nymetro/news/people/columns/intelligencer/12023/ (accessed 10 August 2008).

33. Lois Smith Brady, "Vows: Colleen Saidman and Rodney Yee," *New York Times*, 7 January 2007, http://www.nytimes.com/2007/01/07/fashion/weddings/07Vows.html?_r=1&scp=2&sq=%22Yoga+conference%22&st=nyt&oref=slogin (accessed 10 August 2008).

11. BROKEN OM

1. Alex Kuczynski, "Spiritual Balm, at Only $23.95," *New York Times*, 21 October 2001, http://query.nytimes.com/gst/fullpage.html?res=9501EED7133EF932A15753C1A9679C8B63&sec=&spon=&pagewanted=3 (accessed 20 July 2008).

2. D.T. Emerson, "The Work of Jagadis Chandra Bose: 100 Years of mm-Wave Research," National Radio Astronomy Observatory, February 1998, http://www.tuc.nrao.edu/~demerson/bose/bose.html (accessed 20 July 2008).

3. "The Gospel of Non-Possession," http://www.mkgandhi.org/philosophy/nonpossession.htm (accessed 20 July 2008).

4. "Indian Press Lauds Gandhi Decision," BBC News, 19 May 2004, http://news.bbc.co.uk/1/hi/world/south_asia/3727591.stm (accessed 23 July 2008).

5. Deepak Chopra, "The Amorality of the Free Market," *Washington Post*, 28 May 2008, http://newsweek.washingtonpost.com/onfaith/deepak_chopra/2008/05/greed_as_higher_morality_the_g.html (accessed 31 July 2008).

6. Sam, *Life of Osho* (London: Sannyas, 1997), 13, http://www. universallawstoday.com/ebooks/Life%20of%20Osho.pdf (accessed 31 July 2008).

7. Osho, "Yoga: The Alpha and the Omega, Vol 1," 25 December 1973, http://www.messagefrommasters.com/Beloved_Osho_Books/ Yoga_Books/Yoga_The_Alpha_and_the_Omega_Volume_1.pdf (accessed 31 July 208).

8. Janet Maslin, "Movie Review: Ashram (1981)," *New York Times*, 13 November 1981, http://movies.nytimes.com/movie/157300/Ashram/ overview (accessed 31 July 2008).

9. Osho, "Early Talks: 3 June 1969," 96, http://www.scribd.com/doc/ 3206231/Osho-Early-Talks1 (accessed 8 August 2008).

10. Ibid.

11. Sam, *Life of Osho,* 83.

12. Neal Karlen and Pamela Abramson, "Bhagwan's Realm," *Newsweek,* 3 December 1984, 34, http://www.nealkarlen.com/newsweek/bhagwan. shtml (accessed 11 August 2008).

13. Hugh Milne, *Bhagwan: The God That Failed* (New York: St. Martins Press, 1987), 15.

14. Richard K. Rein, "The Daughter of Jonestown Victim Leo Ryan Argues That Her Guru's Sect Is Not a Cult," *People,* 16 February 1981, http://www.people.com/people/archive/article/0,,20078618, 00.html (accessed 21 July 2008).

15. "Rajneeshism," *Hindusim Today,* January 1984, http://www.hinduism today.com/archives/1984/01/1984-01-09.shtml (accessed 21 July 2008).

16. "First Annual World Celebration, 1982—Rajneeshpuram, Oregon," Dialog Center, 27 November 2007, http://www.dc-international. org/index.php?view=article&catid=150&id=415%3Afirst-annual- world-celebration-1982-rajneeshpuram-oregon&option=com_ content&Itemid=41 (accessed 12 August 2008).

17. Neal Karlen, Pamela Abramson, "Bhagwan's Realm," *Newsweek,* 3 December 1984, 34, http://www.nealkarlen.com/newsweek/ bhagwan.shtml (accessed 11 August 2008).

18. Ibid.

19. Sam, *Life of Osho,* 14.

20. Win McCormack, *The Rajneesh Chronicle* (Portland: New Oregon Publishers, 1987), 126, http://www.winmccormack.com/pdf/cult/ rajneesh_chronicles.pdf (accessed 31 July 2008).

21. Sam, *Life of Osho,* 150.

22. Roy Wallis, "Religion as Fun? The Rajneesh Movement" (Belfast: Queen's University), 191–224.

23. James Weaver, "The Town That Was Poisoned" (Congressional Record, 99th Congress, 1985).

24. W. Seth Carus, Bioterrorism and Biocrimes: The Illicit Use of Biological Agents Since 1900" (working paper, February 2001 revision, Center for Counterproliferation Research, National Defense University, Washington, D.C.), 53, http://www.ndu.edu/center counter/Full_Doc.pdf (accessed 4 August 2008).

25. Ibid., 55.

26. Satya Bharti Franklin, *The Promise of Paradise* (Barrytown, NY: Station Hill Press, 1992), 136–37.

27. Carus, "Bioterrorism and Biocrimes," 54.

28. Ibid.

29. Ibid., 56.

30. "Few Followers of Guru Vote," *New York Times,* 9 November 1984, http://query.nytimes.com/gst/fullpage.html?res=990DE6DE1139F93 AA35752C1A962948260 (accessed 4 August 2008).

31. Carus, "Bioterrorism and Biocrimes," 52.

32. Milne, *Bhagwan,* 230–32.

33. Peter H. King, "Departed Aides Accused by Guru of Murder Attempts, Theft of Millions," *Los Angeles Times,* 17 September 1985.

34. Frank Trippett and Linda Kramer, "Blown Bliss," *Time,* 30 September 1985, http://www.time.com/time/magazine/article/0,9171,959970, 00.html (accessed 7August 2008).

35. Swami Atmo Jayakumar, "Osho Speaks on 'Sheela & the Oregon Happenings pt III,'" sannyasworld.com, http://www.sannyasworld. com/index.php?name=News&file=article&sid=633 (accessed 7 August 2008).

36. Richard Green, "Bhagwan Followers Held in Death Plot," *Seattle Times,* 2 November 1990, http://community.seattletimes.nwsource. com/archive/?date=19901102&slug=1101910 (accessed 7 August 2008).

37. Sam, *Life of Osho,* 155.

38. Sue Appleton, "Was Bhagwan Shree Rajneesh Poisoned by Ronald Reagan's America?" (Pune: Rebel Publishing House, 1988), 24–25.

39. Taylor Clark, "The Red Menace," *Willamette Week,* 10 November 2004, http://wweek.com/story.php?story=5721 (accessed 22 July 2008).

40. Sven Davisson, "The Rise and Fall of Rajneeshpuram," *Ashe: Journal of Experimental Spirituality,* http://www.ashejournal.com/two/davisson. shtml (accessed 22 July 2008).

41. Christopher Hitchens, *God Is Not Great* (New York: Twelve Books, Hachette Book Group, 2007), 198.

42. Sam, *Life of Osho,* 203.

43. Ibid, 234.

44. Lis Harris, "O Guru, Guru, Guru," *New Yorker,* 14 November 1994, 92, http://www.ex-cult.org/Groups/SYDA-Yoga/leave.txt (accessed 25 June 2008).

45. Christopher Calder, "Osho, Bhagwan Rajneesh, and the Lost Truth," 1998, http://home.att.net/~meditation/Osho.html (accessed 27 June 2008).

46. "Oh Kay . . ." The Tao of Cheese, 9 April 2005, http://tao-de-cheese.blogspot.com/2005/04/oh-kay_09.html (accessed 27 June 2008).

47. Joshua Kurlantzick, "The Money Pose," *Mother Jones,* March/April 2005, http://www.motherjones.com/news/dispatch/2005/03/Money_Pose.html (accessed 2 July 2008).

48. Jennifer Claerr, "Bikram Yoga: Hot Yoga or Hot Water?" Associatedcontent.com, 16 October 2007, http://www.associated content.com/article/410634/bikram_yoga_hot_yoga_or_hot_water. html?page=2&cat=5 (accessed 3 July 2008).

49. Neil Chatterjee and Sophie Hardach, "Hollywood Guru Bikram Sells Yoga to 'Ugly Society,'" Reuters India, 3 March 2008, http://in.reuters.com/article/lifestyleMolt/idINSYD24390620080303 (accessed 16 December 2007).

50. Katharine Livingston, "Compilation of Yoga Positions Can Be Protected by Copyright," iplawobserver.com, 19 April 2005, http://www.iplawobserver.com/2005/04/compilation-of-yoga-positions-can-be.html (accessed 3 July 2008).

51. John Pallatto, "Yoga Suit Settlement Beggars Open Source Ideals," Eweek.com, 13 May 2005, http://www.eweek.com/c/a/Enterprise-Apps/Yoga-Suit-Settlement-Beggars-Open-Source-Ideals/ (accessed 8 July 2008).

52. Allison, "Legal Settlement," yoga.com, 18 May 2005, http://www. yoga.com/forums/forums/thread-view.asp?tid=18994&start= 16&posts=30 (accessed 8 July 2008).

53. Bay Guy, "Legal Settlement," yoga.com, 10 May 2005, http://www. yoga.com/forums/forums/thread-view.asp?tid=18994&start=16& posts=30 (accessed 8 July 2008).

INDEX